Dr Chris Idzikowski, BSc, PhD, FBPsS, is Director of the Sleep Assessment and Advisory Service and the Edinburgh Sleep Centre. A leading expert on sleep and its disorders, he has served as Chairman of the British Sleep Society and has been a long-term council member of the Royal Society of Medicine's Sleep Medicine Section. Dr Idzikowski has also sat on the boards of the European Sleep Research Society and the US Sleep Medicine Foundation. He is the author of five books, including *Learn to Sleep Well* (Watkins).

SOUND ASLEEP

THE EXPERT GUIDE TO SLEEPING WELL

CHRIS IDZIKOWSKI

WATKINS PUBLISHING

LONDON

This edition published in the UK and USA in 2013 by
Watkins Publishing Limited, Sixth Floor,
75 Wells Street, London W1T 3QH

A member of Osprey Group

Text Copyright © Chris Idzikowski 2013
Design and typography copyright © Watkins Publishing Limited 2013

1 3 5 7 9 10 8 6 4 2

Designed and typeset by Jerry Goldie Graphic Design

Printed and bound in Italy

A CIP record for this book is available from the British Library

ISBN: 978-1-78028-118-6

www.watkinspublishing.co.uk

Distributed in the USA and Canada by Sterling Publishing Co., Inc.
387 Park Avenue South, New York, NY 10016-8810

For information about custom editions, special sales,
premium and corporate purchases, please contact
Sterling Special Sales Department at 800-805-5489
or specialsales@sterlingpub.com

CONTENTS

Chapter 6: **Sleep disorders – step by step** 137

Chapter 7: **Pills, potions and therapies** 188

AUTHOR'S ACKNOWLEDGMENTS

I'd like to acknowledge simply everyone I've worked with – friends, colleagues, staff, collaborators, students and so on have all contributed to my thinking – but especially my long-suffering editor Judy Barratt and publisher Bob Saxton.

For Hilary
xx

FOREWORD

I've often been asked why I became interested in sleep. After all, for most people sleep is something they barely think about – it comes as a surprise that anyone should devote their working life to understanding it. The short answer is that I don't really remember. I certainly didn't wake up one day and have an extraordinary interest in why I had slept the previous eight, nine, ten hours. I do know, though, that my Latin teacher, my wife, and my late friend and mentor Emeritus Professor Ian Oswald all had something to do with it. Their teaching methods, frank criticism of my work and fascinating insights into the human brain have all inspired me.

Looking after your sleep – and doing it in a way that isn't harmful (by not using sleeping pills or alcohol, for example) is fundamental to your well-being. This book brings together the essence of everything I've learned about sleep in a way that I hope is practical and accessible. My aim has been to give you not only information about the nature of sleep, but also guidance on actions you can take at home to improve your sleep quality. I haven't shied away from the importance of conventional medicine in the treatment of sleep disorders (I'm a scientist, after all), but I hope you'll see that there are lots of ways in which you can enjoy better-quality sleep through simple changes to your lifestyle and by performing simple tasks that promote sleep.

It's important that you work through the book from the beginning. In Chapters 1 and 2, I've offered an understanding of what sleep is and what it does (as far as we know). Information and simple measures will help you to make your own assessments of how well you sleep at the moment and how sleepy you are during the day. By going back to these early assessments when you've read later parts of the book, you can gain a good measure of your progress as you start to implement my techniques and tips for sleep improvement.

Arguably, the critical chapter in the book is Chapter 3 – the chapter on sleep hygiene. A safe building is constructed on deep and solid foundations. Sleep hygiene is the foundation of refreshing sleep. You cannot improve your sleep – at any level – without making good sleep hygiene your priority.

In Chapters 4 and 5, I've looked at some of the specific challenges that we face for our sleep quality at particular times or stages in our lives, as well as in particular circumstances.

If you think you have a sleep disorder, Chapter 6 aims to give practical advice on treatment – I've covered major disorders, as well as some of the more unusual ones. If you have an insomnia, I hope to enable you to make informed choices about your treatment, both at home and with the help of a sleep centre or a doctor.

Finally, in Chapter 7, I've provided a summary of conventional and complementary therapies that are often used to help people overcome sleep problems. Taking a scientific view of what's available, I hope I've offered robust information and advice so that you can choose remedies and therapies that will have actual beneficial effects on your sleep improvement, if you need them.

Overall, I hope this book enables you to better understand the unique nature of your sleep so that you can put in place strategies that work for you. Your physical, emotional and mental well-being rely upon sleeping soundly. I wish you a peaceful night, every night.

Chris Idzikowski, January 2013

CHAPTER 1

SLEEP – AN INTRODUCTION

We know that in the Paleolithic era early man slept on beds of straw, grass, brushwood and pelt. From observing the actions of chimpanzees, we know that our animal ancestors are to this day particular about their sleep. Chimpanzees build nests in trees to keep themselves safe from predators. These nests consist of a mattress lined with soft leaves and twigs. Across time and species, it seems that we don't just need sleep, we need good-quality sleep in comfort and safety.

In this chapter I'll try to answer some fundamental questions about sleep. What is it? What is it for? What are its features? Sometimes the answers are straightforward; often they involve the complex interplay of science, history and educated guesswork. Sleep remains something of a fascinating conundrum, but one that is essential to our existence.

WHAT IS SLEEP?

How would you describe sleep? Is it a period of complete shut-down? Is it total rest? Is it unconsciousness? In fact, sleep is none of these things. Although many people describe sleep as the body's opportunity for stopping, in truth it is one of the most active periods of the day (or, rather, night) for our brain. There is no "shutting down" – two regions of the brain communicate and co-operate to create the state of sleep. In other words, sleep is an active process, not a passive one (and in the morning, the same two regions of the brain work together to create wakefulness). Some scientists think that we burn fewer than a hundred calories less during sleep than we would if we were awake but resting. This undermines the next hypothesis, that sleep is rest: sleep does involve physical rest, but we can rest nearly as effectively without actually sleeping. We aren't unconscious during sleep, because a persistent or loud noise or other physical disturbance will wake us.

One of the most precise ways to describe sleep is to think of it as a temporary severance between the outside world and our perception or experience thereof. At the precise moment of sleep, connections between our brain and our senses virtually cease to function. During sleep we can't really hear, taste, smell, feel touch, or see (except in our dreams). Another feature of sleep is that we can be woken from it (it is a reversible state). During dreaming sleep our limbs are immobilized in order that we can't "act out" our dreams.

In physiological terms, sleep is a period of distinct cycles and stages. An adult with healthy sleep each night goes through four or five sleep cycles (see pp.20–21), each demarcated by an unnoticed moment of wakefulness. Every one of those sleep cycles is itself made up of five stages of sleep – until recently thought of as drowsiness, light sleep, two periods of deep sleep and REM (or dreaming) sleep (these stages have now been reclassified; see p.19). Sleep is triggered when two particular regions of our brain communicate with one another. We'll go into which later, but the process is rather like two conductors trying to conduct a single orchestra to play the perfect tune. When they succeed and the instruments play in harmony, we fall asleep easily. As long as no one steps out of time or tune, we stay asleep. When the instruments are out of kilter, our sleep may not be restful. When this problem persists, we say we have a sleep disorder.

WHAT IS TIREDNESS?

Tiredness comes in many guises. The most common form of tiredness is the form we should all feel at the end of the waking day – a general

SLEEP SCIENCE

WHY DO WE NEED SLEEP?

Evidence suggests that sleep is an important part of maintaining clear waking brain function. We know, for example, that people who are sleep-deprived react more slowly, and have impaired thinking skills and concentration and a poorer memory. Trying to drive when you haven't had enough sleep is like driving under the influence of alcohol. Without sleep, moreover, we may develop poorer physical health. High blood pressure, obesity (and the health issues that go with it, such as heart disease) and stress or anxiety are all common in people who suffer from insomnia or other sleep disorders that severely impair the quality of their sleep.

However, some studies suggest that complete rest, even in a waking state, is almost as restorative to the body and mind as sleep itself. Furthermore, some muscles of the body (such as the heart and diaphragm) continue to work throughout sleep, again suggesting that sleep isn't for resting muscles. On the other hand, we know that all living things, including plants, "go to sleep" for periods of time in the 24-hour day; and that animals with a faster metabolism (meaning that they burn energy more quickly) need more sleep than those with a slower metabolism. We know that the urge to sleep can become overwhelming (fighting sleep takes enormous effort, and eventually sleep will win), even more so when we're ill and need to get better. Most crucially of all, evolution has not phased out sleep. So, if recuperation and restoration are not what sleep is for, and yet sleep is to all intents and purposes "involuntary", why do we need it? Unfortunately, science is still searching for the definitive answer – if indeed there is one. For now, we have to be content simply in accepting that nature intended us to sleep, and that the better quality sleep we can attain, the better our health and well-being and our enjoyment of our waking life.

fatigue that puts us in mind that it's time to go to bed. This is a perfectly normal part of daily life. In itself, it may come as a feeling of mental tiredness (a long day at the office, which makes you feel sleepy), or physical tiredness (an active day hiking, cycling or gardening or doing physical work) – neither of which is a problem, as long as you feel refreshed again after a rest or ideally a good night's sleep.

However, prolonged tiredness or tiredness that prevents you from functioning normally during the day may be a symptom of illness, or even an illness in itself. According to the Royal College of Physicians, a staggering one in ten people in the UK report feeling "tired all the time" and the problem is especially acute among women. If you feel that there's no relief from your feelings of tiredness, you need to investigate what this might mean. Have a look at the box on pages 6–7 and see if any of the prompts apply to you – and then take appropriate action, which of course begins with making sure that your sleep is as healthy and restorative as it can be.

WHAT IS DREAMING?

Austrian psychoanalyst Sigmund Freud (1856–1939) claimed that dreams were the mind's way to release pent-up desires or forbidden thoughts. His contemporary the Swiss genius Carl Jung (1875–1961) believed they formed an expression of our "collective unconscious". He described this as the pool of symbolic archetypes that is identical to all people in all cultures and is distinct from the "personal unconscious", which is the mind's mapping of our own unique experiences.

However, since Freud and Jung put forward their theories, sleep researchers have tried to explain dreaming in rather more scientific terms. Put together a simple electric circuit to light a bulb, but overload the power with too many batteries and the bulb will not light. Our minds are rather like that. During the day, the brain is bombarded with information – from our senses and our learning – for us to process and store. Overload the brain, and we might feel befuddled, exhausted or even unwell. In the 1990s sleep experts considered the possibility that our dreams crucially help the brain to make sense of the overload, sifting through and ordering all the millions of fragments of data we process every day – a sort of unravelling and filing of everything that's on our mind so that the mind itself can work.

This certainly seems to be the case when we look at the physical evidence for dreaming. We think that dreams occur mainly during a specific phase of sleep, known as REM – or Rapid Eye Movement – so-called because the eyes flick back and forth beneath our eyelids as we sleep. More recent research into the nature of REM has suggested that far from being a "light-hearted" break in the serious business of deep sleep, this phase must be essential to our well-being. When human beings are deprived of REM sleep, the body compensates for that deprivation by having extended periods of REM as soon as it can. If REM didn't matter, why would the body or brain try at the soonest opportunity to catch up on the deficit? We still don't fully understand why REM is significant, nor what dreams do exactly, but we can conclude that both seem to be an essential function of a healthy mind.

The characteristics of dreams

There are innumerable ways in which we could describe our dreams, but to the scientific mind there are three main characteristics that are unique to dreaming. First, we're in temporary paralysis during our dreams in order that we can't act them out. Second, we rarely ever dream that we're someone else, even if our dreams are fantastical. Finally, our dreams are fragmented, whereas life is continuous.

Then there's the question of whether or not dreams have meaning. I think this is a matter that entirely depends upon your point of view. Since time immemorial there have been those – scientists such as Sigmund Freud among them – who have believed firmly that dreams unearth deep messages from our unconscious, helping us to make sense of past events or anxieties in our lives. I think that dreaming is a time when you become aware of how your brain is processing infor-mation. For example, teeth probably mean work to a dentist, but they may symbolize death to someone looking to interpret their dreams by traditional associations. So, do your dreams have meaning? Yes, if you believe they do.

SLEEP CLINIC

Why am I tired all the time?

In order to work out what might be causing your prolonged tiredness, you need to consider whether or not the tiredness is mental, physical, a result of your lifestyle or sleep issues, or a combination of all of these factors. Although some of the following common causes of prolonged tiredness may seem alarming – don't panic! Think carefully about what's going on in your life, follow the advice in this book to improve the quality of your sleep, and if your symptoms persist talk to your doctor. If neither of you can find a cause for your ongoing tiredness, it doesn't improve, and it has lasted for over six months, the tiredness is more accurately described as fatigue, and you may have Chronic Fatigue Syndrome. Your doctor will advise you on how to manage this condition.

Mental and emotional causes
- anxiety
- depression
- bereavement
- stress, pressure or too much to do at work or at home

Physical causes
- being overweight
- being underweight
- anaemia (iron deficiency)
- diabetes
- glandular fever, or other glandular illness
- chronic illness, such as cancer or heart disease
- underactive thyroid
- muscular illness, such as multiple sclerosis
- immune conditions, including allergies and HIV

- recovery from an operation or other illness
- certain medical treatments

Lifestyle causes
- anything that disrupts the quality of your sleep, such as drinking too much alcohol or caffeine
- taking too little exercise
- taking too much exercise
- too many demands on your time – or "burning the candle at both ends"

Problems with sleep
- narcolepsy (falling asleep at the "wrong" times)
- sleep apnoea (cessation in breathing as you sleep)
- snoring
- getting too much sleep

SLEEP SCIENCE

TIREDNESS, SLEEPINESS AND FATIGUE

It's important to spell out at this stage the differences between tiredness, sleepiness and fatigue. Tiredness is a general feeling of lethargy. Sleepiness is the feeling of having to fall asleep, an overwhelming urge to close your eyes and drift off. It doesn't result only from tiredness, but a combination of tiredness, posture, what you're doing at any particular time and the environment that you're in (for example, you're more likely to feel sleepy in a warm room than in one that's cool). Fatigue is prolonged tiredness or excessive sleepiness and is characterized by an inability to function properly at a physical or mental level during waking hours.

HOW MUCH SLEEP DO YOU NEED?

Is there such a thing as the "right" amount of sleep? What's normal, and what signifies that we have a problem? As with so much about sleep research, the answers are not easy to give. What's normal, acceptable and restorative for you might for me seem excessive or too little.

Age, genetics, health, the season, and the amount of racked-up sleep debt all help determine the number of hours of sleep each of us needs. And because no two of us are the same, nor are our sleep needs.

In 2009 a company in Massachusetts launched the Zeo (see box, p.202), a personalized sleep monitor that tells you how much light, deep and dreaming sleep you've had each night. For sleep researchers the Zeo is invaluable because it's enabled us to see what an "average" night's sleep is like over a large cross-section of the population (albeit people willing and able to buy the gadget, which at the time of publication is available for between $100 and $200). The readings from almost ten thousand Zeo participants tell us that the average American sleeps 6.8 hours a night, with six percent clocking up fewer than six hours of sleep a night and 12 percent having eight hours or more.

So, does that mean that around seven hours sleep a night is what we should aim for? Perhaps. In order to provide guidelines, experts have agreed that healthy adults need between seven and nine hours sleep. Teenagers need one to two hours more a night; and newborns under two months old should sleep between 12 and 18 hours in every 24. The sleep needs of people aged 65 and over naturally decrease, although there is much speculation as to why, including the consideration that certain medications may disrupt sleep.

As ever, this information is relevant only in light of your uniqueness. Although seven hours might suit your partner, you might need closer to nine. In this book, I've assumed that you're aiming to sleep for eight hours a night, but do adjust my advice in light of your own needs.

YOU AND YOUR SLEEPINESS

Sleepiness is a basic "physiological needs" state. You might compare it to feeling hungry or thirsty. In a different way to hunger and thirst,

SLEEP SCIENCE

TOO MUCH AND TOO LITTLE SLEEP

The dangers of having too little sleep, and the conditions associated with too little sleep, are well-publicized, but less well known are the adverse effects and associations of too much sleep. The lists below clearly set out the effects of both. Notice that some of the effects are the same in both categories.

Effects of or associated with too little sleep
• Poor concentration, memory and vigilance
• Sleepiness, tiredness, fatigue, irritability, weariness
• Increased risk-taking, suggestibility
• Weight-gain
• Depression
• Poor immune health
• Increased risk of diabetes and morbidity
• Increased mortality

Effects of or associated with too much sleep
• Obesity
• Back pain
• Headaches
• Depression

though, the less good-quality sleep you have, the greater your sleepiness, not only when you're about to go to bed, but at other times, too.

How sleepy you feel over the course of the day will depend upon all sorts of factors, including your general health, your age and what's going on around you. If you're stimulated and distracted, it can (up to a point) be quite easy to cast aside sleepiness and work through it.

If you're bored or doing something monotonous, sleepiness is harder to ignore. The elderly often feel sleepy between two and three o'clock in the afternoon, our "natural" siesta; while young adults, commuting from work on their way home, often report feeling sleepy as they drive.

In this respect, sleepiness is dangerous – but not only for your safety while driving a car. It can also affect your critical thinking and memory.

There are three main factors that affect daytime sleepiness:
- The duration of your nighttime sleep (how long you've slept during the night).
- The quality of your nighttime sleep (how well you've slept).
- The circadian time (the time of day).

Measuring sleepiness

In 1990, Dr Murray Johns, the founder of the Sleep Disorders Unit at Epworth Hospital in Melbourne, Australia, devised the "Epworth Sleepiness Scale" (ESS) in order to assess the daytime situations in which clients at his sleep clinic were most likely to feel an overwhelming desire to nod off. He asked his clients to score eight potentially sleep-inducing scenarios on a rising scale of zero to three – with zero indicating that the client wouldn't feel sleepy in that situation and three indicating that the client would almost certainly nod off.

The scenarios Dr Johns gave were: sitting reading; watching TV; sitting inactive in a public place; being a passenger in a car for an hour without a break; lying down to rest in the afternoon; sitting talking; sitting quietly after an alcohol-free lunch; and driving, but being stopped for a few minutes in traffic. If his patients scored nine or more, he took that to be a good indicator that they *might* in fact have a sleep disorder. He assessed that healthy sleepers scored around five.

Measuring fatigue

If the ESS measures general levels of sleepiness, the Fatigue Severity Scale (FSS), developed by Dr Lauren Krupp of New York State University, estimates levels of weariness. Initially created to assess fatigue in patients with multiple sclerosis and the auto-immune condition lupus, the scale is now used to assess likelihood of a sleep disorder. Patients are asked to rate statements relating to how fatigued they feel in certain situations. For example, on a rising scale of one to seven for each, do you feel that fatigue interferes with: your family and work time? Your sustained physical functioning? Your general functioning? And your ability to carry out your responsibilities? Similarly, is fatigue brought on by exercise? Does it affect your levels of motivation? And does it force you to shorten periods of activity? Totting up your score for each, a total of twenty or more suggests you need to take action.

There are lots of online resources that enable you to take the ESS or the FSS, or tests like them. Or, alternatively you can simply score your responses to the scenarios as I've given them here. Over the course of this book, I'll show you ways in which you can considerably improve those scores, which itself means that you'll have improved the quality of your sleep.

CHAPTER 2

THE SCIENCE OF SLEEP

Sleep has fascinated thinkers and philosophers since ancient times. However, the science of sleep – the analytical measurement of this crucial physical state – is still in its relative infancy. In fact, in terms of modern research, sleep science has been around for only about fifty years (that's not to say that others, centuries before, hadn't tried to explain sleep). In this chapter I introduce you to some of the most influential sleep researchers past and present and highlight the contributions they've made to our understanding of sleep. Then I delve deeper into the science of sleep – from what happens to the brain and body as we sleep, to the cycles of sleep and the nature of dreaming.

SCIENTISTS OF SLEEP

Around 350BCE the Greek philosopher Aristotle recorded his thoughts on the nature of sleep and sleeplessness. He concluded, for example, that "sleep is, in a certain way, an inhibition of function, or, as it were, a tie, imposed on sense-perception, while its loosening or remission constitutes being awake." By looking at humans and animals, Aristotle realized that when we sleep our acknowledgment of the senses ceases to function and in this way at least sleep is different from wakefulness.

However, it wasn't until almost two millennia later that scientific investigations into the nature of the brain, as well as into the nature of sleep, made discoveries that now influence the way we think about sleep and wakefulness. In 1842, Edward Binns published *The*

Anatomy of Sleep, the content of which is elucidated by its subtitle, "The art of procuring sound and refreshing slumber at will." Binns mooted that sleep was an active process over which we have some control, rather than a passive one resulting merely as a consequence of tiredness. He believed that human beings could exert influence over sleep by removing all stimulation.

After Richard Caton, a British scientist working in the late 19th century, had attached electrodes to the scalps of animals, establishing that there was electrical activity in the brain, others were able to make great advances in sleep research. In the 1920s the German psychiatrist Hans Berger became the first to reveal that the human brain operated on a number of different electrical frequencies, which he recorded, calling the readings electroencephalograms (EEGs). Crucially for sleep science, he demonstrated that the brainwaves active in the human brain during sleep were different from those associated with wakefulness, although it was several years before anyone believed him.

Around the same time that Berger was making EEGs in Germany, Professor Nathaniel Kleitman, a Russian-born American psychologist, regarded by many as the founder of modern sleep research, was conducting experiments on himself and others to find more evidence for the nature of sleep. He spent periods of time underground, living in Mammoth Cave, Kentucky, to establish what happened to the body when it was forced to exist in perpetual darkness. He found that the body works on a circadian rhythm – a 24-hour cycle – which remains more or less constant whatever the light conditions of our environment.

However, Kleitman's ambitions went beyond wanting to establish that our body doesn't need light and dark in order to follow its natural rhythms. He wanted to challenge what had become the accepted wisdom that sleep was a single, linear state of rest. He proved instead that, as in fact Aristotle had believed centuries before him, sleep was the obverse side of the same coin as wakefulness – that the two were both mutually exclusive and interdependent; that they complemented one another. The result was perhaps his most famous publication, a book called *Sleep and Wakefulness*, which he published in 1939.

Kleitman, who lectured at the University of Chicago until he was over 100 years old, had two students who helped to put sleep medicine firmly on the clinical map. The first, Eugene Aserinsky, with Kleitman, established that REM sleep existed and that it had a connection with dreaming. However, it was another student, William Dement, who examined the connection in detail, firmly concluding that dreaming happens during REM sleep and publishing his findings in 1958.

Back in Europe, Michel Jouvet, a French neurologist and academic, dug deep into Dement's discoveries about the links between dreaming and REM sleep. He went one step further, establishing through a series of experiments on cats that many muscles of the body go into a state of paralysis during REM sleep in order that we can't act out our dreams. He called REM sleep a "paradoxical" stage of sleep in which the body goes into a strange, independent state of alertness.

From the 1960s onward, sleep research became more accepted as a branch of medicine, especially following French neurologist Henri Gastaut's identification of sleep apnoea (see pp.171–4). We still have much to learn, but the work of these scientists makes the job of under-standing sleep and treating its problems that much better informed.

RHYTHMS OF THE DAY AND NIGHT

Almost every living thing – including plants and animals and every individual cell in the body – has a 24-hour rhythm that sees it go through periods of activity and inactivity, fast metabolism and slow metabolism, growth and maintenance. We don't know for certain why this internal 24-hour rhythm has evolved, but presumably it's because that's the daily cycle of the Earth as it turns on its axis while orbiting the Sun. We do know that humans have a specific bundle of between forty and eighty thousand brain cells that act as this internal metronome – it's call the suprachiasmatic nucleus and is located in the hypothalamus at the base of the brain.

Rhythms that are attuned to the earthly 24-hour cycle of day and night are called circadian rhythms (from the Latin *circa*, meaning "about", and *dies*, meaning "day"). Our sleep–wake cycle isn't the only circadian rhythm we have – our oxygen consumption, urine output,

SLEEP SCIENCE

BODY TEMPERATURE AND SLEEP

Your average body temperature is 37°C (98.6°F), and although many people think this is constant, actually over the course of the day and night body temperature undergoes a circadian rhythm that sees tiny fluctuations above and below the average of approximately 0.5°C (slightly less than 1°F). In a healthy adult, body temperature is at its highest around 11pm. After this peak, it begins to fall, and this is one of the triggers that we think tell the body that it's time to sleep. Body temperature reaches its lowest point at around 4am. In the 1990s researchers at Cornell University, New York, conducted an experiment in a carefully controlled environment on 44 healthy adults aged between 19 and 82 years old to try to measure the correlation between temperature and our ability to fall asleep. They found that without any external distractions it took less than 45 minutes for participants to fall asleep once their body temperature had begun to come down. The results suggest that the best time for dropping into slumber is when body temperature is falling at its fastest. For this reason, sleep specialists recommend having a hot bath about 90 minutes before you try to sleep. Then, when you get out of the bath, your body temperature falls rapidly. You should also keep your bedroom relatively cool (see pp.45–9).

muscle strength and, crucially for sleep, body temperature are just some of the other human functions that operate on a 24-hour clock. Think about your own performance over the course of a day. Perhaps you feel more mentally alert in the morning, and more physically able later. Interestingly, many World Records are set when athletes compete in the evening, when physical strength peaks.

In order to be classed as a circadian or biological rhythm, a cycle needs to persist even without external triggers. Nathanial Kleitman

MELATONIN AND YOUR BIOLOGICAL CLOCK

Your pineal gland, a pea-sized structure that lies in the middle-front of your brain, is your body's main source of the hormone melatonin. This hormone – sometimes called the vampire hormone – is secreted when darkness begins to fall. Artificial light prevents the pineal gland from beginning production of melatonin and delays the onset of sleep. Once darkness has fallen, melatonin levels continue to rise, peaking between 3 and 4am. Secretion stops altogether as dawn breaks. Crucially, melatonin does not induce sleep in itself – rather it's a regulator for your biological clock, making sure you sleep during darkness and wake with the light.

proved that the sleep–wake cycle was inbuilt when he spent three months underground without any natural light (see p.13). However, it's important that the rhythms are able to be reset (they are what is known as "entrainable") by exposure to external stimuli, such as light and heat – and this is how we cope with, for example, time zones. Finally, the rhythms must repeat once every 24 hours and they must retain their pattern of repetition regardless of the outside temperature.

The biological clock needs to synchronize with day and night. Anything that helps it get in step is called a *zeitgeber* and the most important zeitgeber we have is light. It's probably for this reason that the suprachiasmatic nucleus sits over the optic nerve, through which the retina of the eye transmits the transitions from light to dark and back again, to the brain. White light is a combination of all the colours of the spectrum. Scientists have discovered that, when it hits the back of the eye, the blue light part of the spectrum strongly activates its own branch of the optic nerve, straight to the suprachiasmatic nucleus. It bypasses the area of the brain that *slowly* perceives dawning light, and triggers the brain to begin dealing with light information, and set up its rhythms accordingly, before you actually perceive the light itself.

SLEEP SCIENCE

LARKS AND OWLS

Like most things in nature, your biological clock is unlikely to be 24-hour perfect – it usually runs slower. If it runs faster, you may wake a little earlier than average and feel bright-eyed and bushy-tailed almost instantly. If that sounds like you, you're known as a *lark*. If your biological clock runs slower, you'll want to be up late into the night, but find getting out of bed in the morning a terrible chore. In which case, you're an *owl*. You might find that you need to tailor your working life to suit your natural preferences: larks might find nightshifts hard to cope with; while early-morning shifts would not suit owls. It's also important to remember that it's not necessarily when you go to sleep or for how long you sleep you need to change to feel more refreshed – but the quality of your sleep once it's begun.

THE BRAINWAVE REVOLUTION

Hans Berger established the existence of brainwaves in the 1920s. He attached electrodes to his subjects' heads (see p.13) and called the recordings electroencephalograms (EEGs). He realized that there was more than one type of brainwave present in the human brain, which led to his identifying and naming "alpha waves" (also known as Berger's waves). Alpha waves are oscillations in the electrical activity of the brain that vary at a rate of between 8 and 12 cycles per second (known as Hertz, or Hz), and Berger noticed that this happens when we're awake, but resting with our eyes closed. He then immediately went on to identify "beta waves" – oscillations of between 12 and 30Hz – which he said occur when we're actively thinking or concentrating.

Since Berger made his discoveries, there has been a brainwave revolution. Berger's revelations were spot on, but they were only the tip of the iceberg. Below is a description of each brainwave type, from the fastest to the slowest, as we understand them.

Beta waves

Among the most frantic brainwaves are beta waves – the more intense our active thought processes, confusion, concentration or stress, the faster the beta-wave oscillations. Beta waves characterize wakefulness and are rarely present during sleep.

Alpha waves

Far from there being only one type of alpha wave, scientists now believe that there are in fact at least three types. The first, as Berger identified, occurs when we're in a state of calm rest, but not asleep or even tired. The second occurs during REM sleep, when alpha waves are emitted from a different part of the brain to those of wakefulness. No one understands fully yet why alpha waves occur during REM sleep, although presumably this has something to do with the fact that REM sleep is usually when we're dreaming. The third type of alpha wave is known as the alpha-delta and it occurs when we're in non-dreaming sleep when there should be no alpha waves at all – it's just that they "intrude" on the delta waves of sleep (see below). Alpha-delta intrusion is associated generally with sleep disorders, and one study published in 2011 has suggested that it may be particularly prevalent in people who suffer from depression (see pp.185–7).

Theta waves

Slow theta waves occur at 4 to 7Hz and indicate a deep state of relaxation, such as you might experience during meditation. They also occur as we drift off to sleep, becoming interspersed among the alpha waves that we experience as we close our eyes and relax. During this brief period between sleep and wakefulness, you might experience strange sensations and hallucinogenic-type visions that characterize a state known as "hypnogogia" (see box, p.21).

Delta waves

The slowest brainwaves that we know about are called delta waves, and it's these brainwaves that characterize deep sleep (although very adept yogis might be able to experience them during meditation, too).

They oscillate at frequencies of between 0 and 4Hz. Interestingly, delta waves occur most frequently in newborn babies, tailing off in their prevalence as we grow older, so that some people over the age of 75 have little delta-wave activity in their brains at all. What happens to the delta brainwaves as we age is still subject to much medical debate but it's certainly not true to say that these over-75s don't experience any deep sleep at all – they do, it's just that we don't quite know how.

CYCLES AND STAGES OF SLEEP

In order to understand how to improve your sleep quality you need to have a broad overview of what happens to your brain during sleep. Sleep is not a one-dimensional state. From the moment sleepiness takes over, you begin a journey through several cycles and several stages.

Ninety minutes

All healthy adults live their lives in perpetual cycles of roughly 90 minutes each, even during waking hours. During sleep, however, these 90-minute cycles are made up of distinct stages, plus REM (or dreaming) sleep. How many stages there are depends whether we're using the old system of sleep classification, or the new one described by the American Academy of Sleep Medicine (AASM) in 2007.

New classifications

Until recently, sleep had been divided into five stages, beginning with drowsiness (Stage One sleep), and moving through light sleep (Stage Two), and two stages of deep sleep (stages Three and Four), and then REM sleep. Under the new system, sleep is instead separated into two major categories – N for non-REM sleep and R for REM sleep. N sleep is sub-categorized as N1, N2 and N3. N1 and N2 are equivalent to Stage 1 and Stage 2 in the old system, while N3 combines the old stages Three and Four, the deepest levels. For simplicity, in other parts of this book, I'll refer simply to **deep** sleep (N3), **light** sleep (N2), **drowsy** sleep (N1) and **dreaming** sleep (R) – unless I need to use the specific classifications for clarity.

A full sleep cycle

A complete adult sleep cycle lasts 90 minutes (and sometimes up to 100 minutes) and we go through roughly four or five of these cycles in a healthy night's sleep. Sleep starts as N sleep. Measuring the onset of this is very difficult, because it's impossible to know at what precise moment we drop from drowsiness into proper slumber. Even when subjects have electrodes attached to them and their brainwaves are measured on an EEG machine, we can't really tell at what exact point wakefulness turns into sleep. We do know, though, that during this time – when we're crossing the threshold into sleep – we might experience dream-like hallucinations that appear at once real and fantastical. This state is known as hypnagogia (a similar state, called hypnopompia, happens as we wake up; see box, opposite).

All of this is characteristic of N1-type sleep, and once we go through this we arrive at N2 sleep, in which the alpha brainwaves give way to theta waves, which may be interspersed by "sleep spindles" and "K complexes". Each of these is a special kind of brainwave that heralds the movement into N2 sleep. Sleep spindles are so called because an EEG chart shows them as a rapid burst of lines. We're still not really sure what their purpose is, but some research indicates that they improve our ability to learn – the more sleep spindles you experience during a sleep episode, the more you're able to take on new information when you wake up. However, why they should occur at this point, as you're entering N2 sleep remains a mystery.

K complexes, on the other hand, are high-voltage bursts of brain activity (they show as extreme peaks and troughs on an EEG graph). Researchers think that they help to prevent you waking during this early part of your sleep cycle by dumbing down your response to noise or other external stimuli. (Interestingly, K complexes will let pass through any "essential" noise – such as someone calling your name, or the sound of your own baby crying – so that you wake up.)

Finally, theta waves become interspersed with delta waves, the slowest brainwaves of sleep. Have you ever felt disoriented or confused when someone has woken you from sleep? Perhaps they've then told you that they were trying to wake you for a while? If so, you were

SLEEP SCIENCE

HYPNAGOGIA AND HYPNOPOMPIA

In the moments before sleeping and before waking, you may experience dream-like hallucinations. Respectively, these periods in your sleep cycle are called hypnagogia and hypnopompia. When you think back to your experiences of falling asleep, perhaps you remember feeling as though you were falling, or you spun out a conversation you wish you'd had during the day – the conversation you have in your head may seem at once realistic and imaginary. These are the sorts of hypnagogic experiences that people report when woken from the precipice of sleep.

In the morning, the process of reconnecting with the world, including the sudden influx of sensory information, can cause feelings of confusion as you separate the associations and random images of your dreams from the certain sensations of reality. In a sense hypnopompia is your waking brain's way to try to force the logic of the real world (which you're waking up to) onto the illogic of your dream world (which you're leaving behind). The result is the feeling of disorientation you have as you come out of sleep.

far into N3-type sleep. This slow-wave sleep is the deepest sleep we have, and interestingly it's the time when most people experience night terrors or sleepwalking.

After a period in N3 sleep, we complete the 90-minute sleep cycle by "rising" again to N2 (light) sleep and then entering a period of R (REM/dreaming) sleep. During R, the body undergoes a temporary paralysis to prevent us from acting out our dreams. In addition, the brainwave frequencies become similar to those of wakefulness (alpha and beta waves), which suggest that the brain is active – perhaps the strongest indication we have that we dream during R.

As the period of R draws to a close, we experience a momentary waking before beginning the next 90-minute cycle of the night. Most people don't even notice that they've risen to the surface of sleep before descending again into a new phase.

How long do we spend in each stage?

Although each sleep cycle lasts roughly 90 minutes, the lengths of time we spend in each stage of sleep within each cycle are not the same. Over the course of the night, periods of N3 sleep shorten (our longest period of deep sleep occurs during the first sleep cycle), while periods of R sleep lengthen, until our last sleep cycle is made up mostly of N2 (light) and R sleep. Overall, we spend up to five percent of the night in N1 (drowsy) sleep; up to 50 percent of the night in N2 (light) sleep and up to 25 percent of the night in N3 (deep) sleep. Around 20 percent of the night is spent in R sleep.

Perfect cycles, perfect sleep

Healthy sleep follows these patterns more or less to the letter. As long as nothing upsets them, sleep is restorative and restful. However, so much in life conspires to send sleep out of kilter. The techniques in this book aim to put all your sleep stages and cycles back in sync.

THE SCIENCE OF DREAMING

We learned at the end of the last section that we spend around 20 percent of our sleeping life in dreaming (R) sleep. Although we do dream in other stages of sleep, most of our dreams occur while we experience REM, so if we're trying to understand the scientific nature of dreaming, R sleep seems to be the obvious place to start.

R sleep is triggered by electrical impulses from a distributed network of neurons located in the brainstem, which sits on top of the spinal column. Slightly higher is the pons, a small area of the brain (measuring about 2.5cm/1in) that's responsible for shutting off the nerves that feed into the spinal column. This causes the temporary paralysis we associate with R sleep. Higher still in the brain is an area called the thalamus. This filters messages to the cerebral cortex, the learning centre of the brain, where we do all our thinking and sorting.

CAN I CONTROL MY DREAMS?

I'm not a great believer in dreams as a reflection of our hidden thoughts and desires. I do, however, think that we have the ability to control our dreams. When we become aware of our dreams, we're said to be lucid dreaming, a term coined by Dutch psychiatrist Frederik van Eeden (1860–1932). During lucid dreams the brain displays greater beta-wave activity, the frantic waves most clearly associated with wakefulness, and it's at this time that some people can become aware of and then take control of their dreams. Some people, it seems, are naturally able to dream lucidly, taking very little time to become quite adept at it; while others may have to learn techniques, and apply these techniques for several months before they achieve lucidity and control. If you're interested in being able to control your dreams, on pages 133–5 I've set out several methods that have been shown to work.

During R sleep our eyes move beneath our eyelids and our breathing quickens and becomes more shallow and irregular. Our heart rate and blood pressure increase, and men have erections, while vaginal secretions increase in women. R sleep must be important to our well-being because we know that we catch up on it as a matter of priority if we don't get enough of it on a particular night. So does this mean that dreams are essential for our well-being, too?

During R sleep we consolidate information. We know this because one study showed that participants who were deprived of R sleep after learning a new skill had impaired ability to perform that new skill when they woke up. A study conducted at Harvard Medical School and published in 2008 supports the notion that dreaming is a representation of the real and relevant in our lives. The sleep researchers discovered that, far from dreaming about events buried within the vaults of our childhood memories, we're more likely instead to dream about events that have happened in the last seven days. Furthermore, many of the participants in the Harvard study claimed that the events that triggered their dreams were not those they would have considered to be significant for their daily lives, despite the fact that the brain had picked them out as needing attention during sleep. (Interestingly, the same group indicated that most of their dreams were negative.)

We might conclude, then, that far from being some sort of fragmented, otherworldly existence, or indeed the "royal road to the unconscious" as Freud suggested, most of our dreams (at least those associated with R sleep) are essential to or a by-product of learning consolidation, and memory. They help to sort and process actual events, even those we think are unimportant, filing them so that they become an integral deposit in our memory bank.

Other research suggests explanations along similar lines, but rather than day-to-day events being the triggers for dreams, our emotions become the dream-weavers. In this theory, scientists think that we need to consolidate highly emotive or traumatic events into our memory bank so that these events no longer feel exceptional or stressful. For example, if you got stuck in an elevator, you might feel claustrophobic or frightened. Over the subsequent nights, elevators themselves *may* feature in your dreams, but it's more likely that the *emotions* you had when you were stuck are reflected in a different set of dream circumstances. Perhaps, then, your feelings of claustrophobia instead trigger a dream about drowning – or another situation in which you feel panic and that you can't breathe. During the dream scenario, your mind processes the emotion and files it away appropriately in your memory bank. It may take more than one night to stop having claustrophobic dreams, but eventually they subside. Scientists moot that at this point you have rationalized the traumatic elevator experience and filed it away with other events that you've already dealt with.

THE GENETICS OF SLEEP
Although we can influence most aspects of our lives, from our fitness to our mood, there's an element of us that's genetic – a physiological

imprint inherited from our forefathers that we can't readily alter. Some of the clients I meet are surprised to learn that aspects of our sleep cycles and sleep patterns fall into this category. In the last two decades, sleep research has made considerable advances in understanding how our genetic legacy influences our sleep. How alert we are during the morning or evening (known as "morningness" or "eveningness"), how long we sleep for, the length of time we spend in the stages of sleep, and the patterns of our brainwaves during both dreaming and other stages of sleep have all been shown to be subject to genetic influence.

As you're probably already beginning to grasp, sleep is a complex behaviour and many aspects of it differ considerably from person to person. This is true even when we compare people who are very close in age. Research into identical and non-identical twins has provided us with important clues as to how many of our sleep patterns are determined by upbringing, the environment and our lifestyle and how many are influenced by our genetic make-up.

A quick lesson in genetics

Understanding the human genome is one of the most complex, intricate and fascinating aspects of human biology. Our genetic information is stored in 23 pairs of chromosomes. We inherit one chromosome in each pair from each of our parents. Our chromosomes are made up of DNA (deoxyribonucleic acid) and our genes are special units of DNA. All genes have different strains, or variants, and these are called alleles. For example, the gene relating to eye colour can be subdivided into alleles for both, for example, blue and brown. If you inherit a blue allele from your mother, but a brown one from your father, you'll have brown eyes, because the allele for brown dominates that for blue. To have blue eyes, you must inherit blue alleles from both your parents.

The health of your genes is not constant. All sorts of factors may cause "gene mutation" – when changes in DNA modify your genetic make-up as your cells subdivide. Sunlight, pollution and exposure to bacteria are all causes of gene mutation. Sometimes gene mutations can improve our genes, while at other times they may damage them and cause disease. Or, they may have no effect on our genes at all.

Genes and your biological clock

The most important genetic discoveries relating to sleep have been made by "chronobiologists", scientists who study our biological rhythms. For example, one family of genes, known as the *Period* genes (*PER1*, *PER2* and *PER3*, found on chromosomes 17, 2 and 1 respectively) relate to our 24-hour metabolic and rest–activity rhythms. Scientists have now developed a genetic test for *PER2* to identify whether or not a person's morningness or eveningness is genetically inherited. Another gene, called the *Circadian Locomotor Output Cycles Kaput* (*CLOCK* for short), is central to the control of circadian rhythms, but also regulates our weight, affects our susceptibility to insomnia and can impact our mood. Both *CLOCK* and *PER3* are among several genes that regulate the biological clock in all kingdoms of life – including the plant kingdom. Have you ever wondered what it is that triggers a flower to open its petals to the sun? *CLOCK* and *PER3* provide part of the answer. (Interestingly, *PER3* is also thought to protect the amount of deep sleep you amass during the night.)

Genes, sleepiness and wakefulness

It won't surprise you to learn that there are genes that control your tendencies to sleepiness and wakefulness, too. Adenosine genes (there are several variants) are biological molecules central to the energy transfer that occurs in all cells of the body – and they also promote sleep. In fact, if you drink a cup of coffee and then find you can't sleep, it's probably because the caffeine has "blocked" the messages the adenosine wants to send your brain to make you sleepy (see p.67).

Genes and how long you sleep

Between 17 and 40 percent of your sleep duration is accounted for by your genetic inheritance. One of the most important genes in this process is *PROK1*, which controls the onset of your "biological night" – the window of opportunity during which your biological clock is telling your body it's time to sleep. In people who are naturally long sleepers, the window of opportunity is relatively long; in short sleepers, predictably, it's relatively short. *PROK1* is not the only gene responsible for the number of hours you spend asleep. Recent research has identified another gene, called *ABCC9*, which can dictate sleep need by plus or minus around 30 minutes. One in five people are thought to have this gene, which works by detecting energy levels in the cells of the body and triggers sleep when it senses they are relatively low.

What do genes mean for you?

The study of the genes of sleep is essential to scientific understanding of how sleep works. With each new link we make between sleep and genetics we have the potential to unlock more of the codes of sleep. For you, though, understanding your tendency to be a lark or an owl, accepting that you may need a longer or shorter time in bed and understanding that the environment affects your genes are all important because they help you to tailor your sleep-improvement strategy in line with your biological make-up. For example, if you're naturally a short sleeper, there's little point in trying to force yourself into sleeping longer – you'll only get frustrated. Instead, you need to tune in to your natural rhythm and capitalize on your window of sleep opportunity as well as take steps that improve the quality of your sleep.

A MEMORY FOR SLEEP

I've heard people say that a good night's sleep improves memory. Certainly, a good night's sleep is essential for waking alertness and so learning, but memory – the cognitive embedding of information and experiences – has a rather more complex relationship with sleep.

A little bit about memory

Memory is subdivided into two main types – declarative (itself divided into episodic and semantic memory) and procedural. Declarative memory is our memory of facts and figures, events and occurrences. It provides the storehouse for our personal history (all the events that have happened to us, our episodic memory) and learned data (our semantic memory). Procedural memory, sometimes called "implicit" memory, on the other hand, is our record of how to do things using our motor skills – from doing up buttons to riding a bike or driving a car. The term "implicit" derives from the fact that as we repeat a task, we learn the movements we need to perform it to the point that those movements become automatic – we don't consciously recall the process of how to perform the task, we just get on with it. Declarative memory, by contrast, is "explicit", because it represents knowledge we have to consciously recall when we need it.

It has taken several decades of sleep research for us even to begin to understand the relationship between memory and sleep. It's only really since the discovery of sleep brainwaves and since we've been able to measure them using electrodes that scientists have made any significant breakthroughs. The summary of the discoveries so far is that consolidation of declarative memories appears to occur during slow-wave (deep) sleep, while the consolidation of procedural memories appears to occur primarily during dreaming sleep, when the brainwaves operate at higher frequencies, more akin to the alpha brainwaves of wakefulness.

Declarative memory and your sleep

In order to test the relationship between sleep stages and declarative memory, scientists attach electrodes to participants' scalps to measure the sleeping brain to operate at certain frequencies. Several studies since the early 1990s have shown that declarative memory is improved when the brain tips into slow-wave sleep. During slow-wave sleep, regions of the brain associated with memory and learning, specifically the hippocampus and the neo-cortex, communicate with one another. New information that has been temporarily stored in the hippocampus is transferred to the neo-cortex, where it becomes part of our long-term learning – it's consolidated. The process of transferring information from one place to the other is generally slow – it can take weeks, months or possibly years for full consolidation to occur. In the process, perhaps unsurprisingly, some of the information is lost.

However, if you were thinking that this means you can play facts and figures into your brain as you sleep and expect to wake up with them permanently embedded, you must think again. I know from experience that the process doesn't work: many years ago I tried it in an attempt to learn my Latin vocabulary in time for an examination – it didn't help! It appears (we don't know for sure yet) that new information must have passed into the hippocampus up to at least an hour or so *before* you go to sleep in order for consolidation of that type of memory to take place *during* sleep. If we learn something immediately before sleep onset, or try to learn it during sleep, we tend not to be able to recall the information when we wake up. Think back over your own experience of learning – did you ever drift off during a class or lecture? If you did, it's likely that you had no memory of the last things you were taught just before you fell into sleep. This is because that new information hadn't made it as far as your hippocampus yet.

Getting good amounts of deep sleep is essential for retaining information you've learned over the course of the day. One experiment gave participants two lists of words to memorize on separate occasions. They were asked to recall as many words as possible from the first list on the same day that they had learned them, before having any sleep. They were asked to recall the second list after a period of slow-wave sleep. On average, participants were able to recall five more words after they'd been able to sleep than they could in the test conducted on their ability to learn during a single period of wakefulness. In short, deep sleep appears to be an important aspect of learning consolidation.

Procedural memory and your sleep

During R sleep brainwaves mirror those of wakefulness, appearing as beta, alpha and theta waves. When the word test described above was conducted to reveal any changes to learning during R sleep it showed no difference in the number of words the participants could recall compared with their recall without having had any R sleep. The same was not true for procedural memory tasks. A common experiment to test procedural learning – motor-skill learning – is to teach subjects to draw mirror images. Scientists have found that we're much better at remembering how to draw the mirror image of something if we've had a period of R sleep, than if we've had no opportunity to sleep, or have had the opportunity to enter only other stages of sleep.

Interestingly, procedural memories tend to involve functions that we learn quickly. This is because they relate to our movement "memory" pathways, particularly the action-related synapses (synapses are the gaps between our neurones). During R sleep, the synapses are used again and again, as if the neurons are re-training during sleep. R sleep, then, is essential for quickly remembering new motor skills. Think back to when you learned to ride a bike. Once you could do it, you could do it – you didn't have to re-learn the motor skills needed for bike-riding the next time you tried. Even if you were a bit wobbly, fundamentally, once you'd learned the skill, you'd learned it for ever.

Of course, all this is to dramatically simplify the relationship between memory and sleep. The links are strong, and our understanding of them grows almost weekly. Inevitably, by the time you come to read this, someone somewhere will have already discovered something new about the relationship between the two.

YOUR BODY DURING SLEEP

As we've already seen, sleep is not a one-dimensional, linear resting state. The mind is busy as we sleep – and so is the body.

Hormones and chemicals

Body and brain function is controlled by a complex interplay of nerves and chemicals. Hormones are natural chemicals produced by the body's glands. They're secreted into the blood to give instructions to our cells. For example, the ovaries and testes secrete the hormones oestrogen and testosterone respectively, and these affect the way we grow and function, underpinning many of the physical and behavioural characteristics that make women and men different.

The body does not secrete hormones the whole time – think of the menstrual cycle, which is guided by the rise, fall and interplay of a woman's hormones over the course of a month. Other hormones (in both men and women) are dependent on sleep onset or a particular sleep stage, or are secreted only when it's dark (see box, p.16). Or, they might vary along a 24-hour rhythm irrespective of sleep.

For example, the pituitary gland secretes growth hormone (GH) during the day and during times of stress. However, secretions are at their highest during sleep, and specifically during deep sleep. This is why young children who sleep very badly might be small for their age. The body is brilliant at compensating for insufficient deep sleep (if you don't get enough one night, it will try to make up for it as soon as you next fall asleep), which means that in general we tend to get the right amounts of GH to remain healthy. GH is also implicated in a healthy immune system, in mental well-being and in the ageing process.

The sex hormones, on the other hand, have a more complex relationship with sleep. For a start the secretion of the sex hormones is not constant over the course of our lives; instead it changes according to whether we are, for example, going through puberty or (in women) pregnancy, or whether we're entering old age. In the majority of children, secretion of two of the sex hormones, follicle-stimulating hormone and luteinizing hormone, occurs at the onset of sleep. During puberty the amount secreted at night increases. With the advent of adulthood, the body secretes more of these hormones over the course of the day so that the rate of release is roughly the same both by night and by day. Testosterone, though, which is present in girls as well as boys, seems linked to the first episode of dreaming sleep we experience at night. Lack of sleep appears to dramatically lower levels of testosterone in the blood of young adults, but the levels return to normal as soon as the sleep deficit has been overcome.

Sleep and your nervous system

The human nervous system consists of two main parts: the central nervous system (CNS), which is the brain and nerve tissue in the spine; and the peripheral nervous system (PNS), which is everything else and isn't protected by bone. The brain is the control centre for both systems. The PNS is itself subdivided in two: the somatic nervous system (the nerves that control our muscles) and the autonomic nervous system (ANS), which controls automatic functions such as heartbeat, breathing rate and salivation. Digestion is governed also partly by the ANS, as well as by its own set of nerves – the enteric nervous system.

SLEEP CLINIC
***

What happens to my hormones if I don't get enough sleep?

Persistent sleep deficit has consequences for four main hormones in your body, as follows.

1. Growth hormone (GH) deficit: Growth hormone is essential for your overall health and the body's repair systems and secretion usually peaks during deep sleep. Your body is very good at making up the deficit of the occasional bad night (see p.31), but prolonged deficit forces the body to secrete the hormone at other times to try to repay the debt. However scientists think that, secreted outside deep sleep, the hormone's efficacy is diminished.

2. High cortisol: Cortisol is a stress hormone. If you have a sleep deficit, its levels remain high in the evening (when they should dip), making it harder to fall asleep and creating vicious cycle.

3. Insulin and glucose confusion: During healthy sleep, blood glucose levels rise, so levels of the hormone insulin rise too in order to move excess glucose out of the blood and store it as glycogen in the cells. Lack of sleep impairs the insulin response, leading to rising blood sugar – and potentially diabetes.

4. Too little leptin: The "satiety" hormone, leptin helps us to feel full when our calorie intake has reached appropriate levels. If you have had too little sleep, your leptin secretions may be up to a third lower than healthy sleepers. As a result you may consume roughly 900 calories a day more than you actually need in order to feel full – which can lead to obesity.

As well as our CNS and PNS, we have a set of 12 pairs of cranial nerves, which emerge from the brain rather than the spinal column. Of these 12 pairs, the most important for sleep is the vagus (from the Latin for "wandering") nerve. Once it leaves the brain, this nerve wends its way through the body both controlling organs and passing sensory information from the organs to the brain. Overstimulation of the vagus nerve during wakefulness can make you feel dizzy or may lead to fainting. If you've ever felt wobbly after vomiting or experienced a head rush when you've felt squeamish, those experiences are a result of overstimulation of your vagus nerve. Prolonged overstimulation, which can happen if you're under stress, has a dramatic effect on sleep – reducing levels of dreaming sleep over the course of a night.

Finally, lack of sleep can itself affect the nervous system. Many studies have shown that the ANS is severely disrupted in shift workers, whose biological clocks step out of rhythm with "normal" night and day. Even if you don't work shifts, if you find it hard to get to sleep, or to stay asleep, to the extent that your biological clock starts to tick out of sync, there may be implications for your ANS, and in particular its regulation of the rhythms of your heart. Furthermore, we know that severe lack of sleep may lead to feelings of irritability, wooziness, or being out of touch or even, in extreme cases, feelings of being disconnected from the world. This in itself suggests that sleep is essential for the health of the nervous system – when we don't get enough of it, we feel we might be going slightly mad.

Sleep and your heart

The heart and circulation are controlled by the autonomic nervous system (ANS; see above). The ANS is itself divided up into the parasympathetic and sympathetic nervous systems. Via the vagus nerve, the parasympathetic nervous system slows down the heart and the sympathetic system speeds it up. The heart itself has pacemakers that provide a basic rhythm of around eighty to 100 beats per minute.

The different sleep stages affect the heart in different ways. During N sleep the ANS is relatively stable. With the body at complete rest both physically and mentally, and with no external influences, the heart and breathing become more settled than at any other time. Unfortunately, R sleep upsets this perfect state of equilibrium.

During R sleep the whole ANS is not as well regulated as usual. It's rather like a faulty thermostat – if the thermostat is set at 20°C (68°F), when it's functioning properly it will turn off at 22°C (72°F) and

> ### SLEEP CLINIC
>
> #### *How can I prevent nighttime reflux?*
>
> During the day your saliva neutralizes acid that escapes into the oesophagus before it reaches your throat. At night you produce less saliva, which means that sometimes stomach acid reaches your mouth to cause the burning sensation we know as heartburn or acid reflux. There are several things you can do:
>
> - Lose weight if you're overweight
> - Always eat your evening meal at least three hours before bedtime
> - Sit up straight when you eat
> - Raise the head-end of your bed by placing something under it, such as a couple of books, blocks of wood, or bricks (using extra pillows for your head alone is not as effective)

turn on again at 18°C (64°F). If the electronics go awry, it might turn off at 25°C (77°F) and on again only when it reaches 15°C (59°F). During R, ANS control of our organs is similar – the trigger points for maintaining our organs become looser. Rather than ticking over, the sympathetic and parasympathetic nervous systems experience surges of activity – a sudden braking because the heart has started to beat too fast and a sudden acceleration because it has become too slow.

In a healthy individual this is not much of an issue, but if you suffer from heart or circulatory disease it does become a problem – and is probably why the rates of heart attack during sleep peak after 4am: the later stages of sleep contain the longest periods of R.

Sleep and your digestion

The digestive system is governed by the ANS, as well as its own set of controls, called the enteric nervous system. Although we might think of digestion as beginning in the stomach, actually it begins in the brain before moving to the mouth. At the back of the throat lies the oesophagus, the food pipe that leads to the stomach. The oesophagus is

FEELING FULL AND FEELING SLEEPY

In 1920 one doctor observed that a balloon inserted into the middle of the small intestine and inflated sent the subject to sleep. Although his findings appeared accurate, we now know that it's not the distention of the small intestine that causes the sleepiness, but the contractions that move the food along. We know this because the sleepy effect doesn't happen if the intestine is filled with water instead of solid food. It also looks likely that some of the intestinal hormones are soporific. However, there's still lots to learn about the correlation between feelings of fullness and feelings of sleepiness. In the meantime, if you don't want to feel sleepy at your desk in the afternoon, have a light lunch.

important in sleep terms: at the top of it there's a striated muscle (one that is partly involuntarily and partly voluntarily controlled) called the "cricopharyngeus". This muscle is unusual because, unlike all the other striated muscles in the body, it's not paralyzed during R sleep, so that we can swallow. However, at night we do swallow less, which is good, because each swallow causes a momentary sleep interruption.

Further along the digestive system, in the small intestine, nutrients continue to be absorbed from our day's food, but in general intestinal activity slows down during sleep. Most importantly, the peristaltic waves that usually carry waste into the anal canal run in reverse, keeping waste back and so minimizing our need for the loo in the night. (This is the reason why we often need to go first thing in the morning, when the system reverses again and the night's waste is pushed on.)

Sleep and your immune system

The precise relationship between sleep and immunity is still unclear. We know that fevers tend to be worse at the night. As fever is one of the ways your immune system fights disease, this suggests that sleep provides support for your body's infection-fighting mechanisms. We also know that growth hormone triggers repair in the body during sleep. Furthermore, when we're ill one of the first immune responses is to raise the level of sleepiness, and when we do sleep we spend longer in deep sleep and less time in dreaming sleep than when we're well.

Scientists hypothesize that sleep simply provides a means to enforce physical rest so that available energy can divert to support the body's fight against disease. Furthermore immunizations provide better protection if we have a good night's sleep after the immunization has taken place. So if you're going abroad or are in line for the flu vaccine, do all you can to sleep well on the night after your injection.

CHAPTER 3

SLEEP HYGIENE –
THE DEEP SLEEP CLEANSE

In order to get a good night's sleep, you need to first assess and then address your "sleep hygiene". This isn't just the need to have a wash and to brush your teeth before you go to bed (although that can come into it), it's also making sure that your sleeping environment, your diet and lifestyle and all the things you do in the hours before you go to bed are as conducive as possible to a night of restorative slumber.

This chapter begins with a short self-assessment aimed at evaluating the state of your sleep hygiene right now. Then, we look at each element of the sleep hygiene model, so that one by one I can show you the importance of each and offer practical advice on how to resolve any issues. By the end of the chapter, you'll have all the information you need to optimize your chances of sleep success.

THE SLEEP HYGIENE REVIEW

There's a difference between regularly getting a bad night's sleep and clinical insomnia, which is a chronic, medical condition. Although many people do have some form of insomnia, there are many thousands of others who could improve their sleep simply by improving their sleep hygiene – a set of sleep-related behaviours, activities and cues that prepares babies, children and adults for good-quality sleep. These sleep-enhancing activities and cues are numerous, complex and inter-related. They can be grouped into four categories for consideration: (1) environmental (including temperature, noise and light); (2) scheduling (when you go to sleep and when you wake up); (3) sleep practices (such as having a bedtime routine); and (4) physiological or lifestyle practices (for example, whether and when you exercise, how much alcohol or caffeine you drink, if any, and when you eat your meals).

We don't yet fully understand why good sleep hygiene promotes good sleep, but of all the cues sleep practices are probably the most important. This is because these may help to entrain your 24-hour internal rhythms to your environment (the 24-hour cycle of night and day). Conditioning comes into this, too – the psychological links you make between activities and environments and the promotion of sleep.

The following self-assessment is intended to give you some level of understanding of whether there are simple improvements to your lifestyle, sleep environment and overall well-being that might have a beneficial affect on your sleep quality. The questionnaire isn't meant to be rigorously scientific – it's simply a means for you to see what you're doing right and where you might be going wrong, so that you can effectively follow the advice in the rest of this chapter. Choose the answers that relate most closely to you, then tot up the numbers of As, Bs and Cs you have overall and read the summaries at the end.

About your sleep environment

1. How relaxed do you feel in your bedroom?
   a. Very – it's clutter-free and a place I save for sleep
   b. Moderately, but I sometimes bring work to bed with me, or I occasionally watch TV in bed
   c. Not at all – I have to use the space for working, gaming and watching TV (or any combination), too

2. How warm is your bedroom?
   a. Below 18°C (64.5°F)
   b. Between 18°C (64.5°F) and 23°C (73.5°F)
   c. Over 23°C (73.5°F)

3. How dark is your room when you go to bed?
   a. It's very dark, almost completely black
   b. I sleep with a nightlight, or with moonlight or streetlight
   c. I keep the overhead light, hall light or bedside lamp on

4. How quiet is your bedroom at night?
   a. Completely quiet
   b. Mostly quiet – I'm only ever disturbed by random or unexpected noises
   c. There's street or neighbour noise that regularly disturbs me

5. How comfortable is your bed?
   a. Very comfortable – I rarely wake up with aches and pains
   b. Fairly comfortable, but I occasionally wake up with an ache, particularly if I've slept in a different position
   c. I wake up every morning with pains, but they go away once I've been up for a few hours

About your sleep schedule and practices

Answer the following questions for a typical week, ignoring exceptions.

6. Do you go to bed at the same time every night?
   a. Yes, I'm always in bed at the same time to within 30 minutes
   b. Yes, during my working week, but I tend to stay up later on Friday and Saturday nights
   c. No, my bedtime mostly varies depending upon my workload or whether or not I'm doing something social in the evening

7. Do you get up at the same time in the morning?
   a. Yes, I get up at the same time, even at the weekend
   b. Yes during the working week, but I often lie in at the weekend
   c. No, I get up when I feel like it

8. Do you ever take a daytime nap (that is, a nap at any time before your usual bedtime, even if it's unintentional)?
   a. No, I never nap

b. Yes, but only at the weekends

c. Yes, I take a daytime nap more than twice a week

9. Do you have a bedtime ritual (any sequence of events that you regularly perform just before you go to bed counts as a ritual)?

a. Yes, I have a sequence of activities that I perform before I go to bed and I do these most if not all nights of the week

b. I do, but I often get distracted while I'm going about it and so find myself doing other things, too

c. No, I don't think about the sequence of events before I go to bed – they tend to be random or I just go to bed

10. What makes you decide to go to bed?

a. I feel tired and that's usually at a particular time of night

b. A certain time comes around, and I go to bed then regardless of whether or not I feel sleepy

c. There's nothing on TV or I feel bored, so I go to bed

About your lifestyle

Again, answer these questions in the light of a typical week.

11. Do you take regular exercise (any activity that raises your heart rate a little above its resting rate for at least 30 minutes)?

a. Yes, I exercise at least three times a week for at least 30 minutes

b. Yes, but only when I can fit it in – perhaps once one week and twice or three times the next

c. No, I exercise very rarely or not at all

12. If you exercise, do you generally do it:

a. In the morning?

b. Between midday and 5pm?

c. After 5pm?

13. How close to bedtime do you eat your main evening meal?

a. At least four hours before I go to bed

b. Two to four hours before I go to bed

c. Fewer than two hours before I go to bed

14. How often do you drink coffee, tea or other caffeinated drinks after 2pm?
    a. Never – I drink my last caffeinated drink with my lunch and then lay off for the rest of the day
    b. Less than twice a week, only if I need a pick-me-up in the afternoon
    c. More than twice a week

15. How often do you drink over one unit of alcohol in the evening?
    a. Once or twice a week, or never
    b. Three or four times a week
    c. More than four times a week

16. If you do drink alcohol in the evening, how close to bedtime do you have your last drink?
    a. More than four hours before bedtime
    b. Between two and four hours before bedtime
    c. Less than two hours before bedtime

17. How often do you use your bedroom for anything other than sleep and sex?
    a. Never – my bedroom is my sanctuary
    b. Occasionally – I have a computer in my room/I take my laptop to bed so that I can catch up on some work before I go to sleep if I really need to
    c. Often – I have a TV in my room and always watch TV in bed/ work in my bedroom

18. How often do you go to bed feeling worried or stressed
    a. Very rarely – generally I'm calm when I go to bed
    b. Occasionally, if I've had a particularly difficult week
    c. Frequently – I find it very hard to switch off from the day

What it all means

Mostly As: If you scored mostly As, your sleep hygiene is heading for exemplary! Take a look at the sections where you scored Bs or Cs and address those issues in order to improve your sleep quality. If, after doing this, you still have trouble sleeping, read the chapter on sleep disorders to see if one of them applies to you.

Mostly Bs: You have a relatively good handle on your sleep hygiene, but there are some areas that you could improve. Read the sections that apply to the questions in which you scored Bs and Cs and see what improvements you can make. Also, read the chapter on sleep disorders to rule out whether or not one of these applies to you.

Mostly Cs: It's likely that you could dramatically improve the quality of your sleep by improving your sleep hygiene. Look at the questions for which you scored Cs and read the relevant sections of this chapter to help you improve those areas of your sleep hygiene. Then, tackle the Bs. Be patient – it may take several months for you to see a significant improvement in your sleep quality. If, however, after six months of implementing my sleep hygiene advice you have no improvement in your sleep, consider whether you're suffering from a sleep disorder.

YOUR SLEEPING SPACE

Your sleeping space is for sleep and sex. Nothing else. As soon as you step inside your bedroom, the associations have to be clear. To this end, there are a few "keep out" rules that you'll need to put in place.

Keep out...

... *the TV*

In the UK recent reports estimate that a staggering one in five under-four-year-olds has a television in his or her bedroom; the figures are worse in the USA. We can only assume that if you grow up with a TV in your bedroom, you'll continue to have one into adulthood.

Television is one of the greatest reasons for our ignoring the urge to fall asleep on a typical day. If the TV is moved into the bedroom, the ease of having it on while you get ready for bed – and then keeping it on once you're in bed – means that you may overlook your body's sleep signals, or even fight them off for as long as possible.

In addition, TV can act as a stimulant, encouraging the brain to keep active, processing pictures and stories. Have you ever watched an action movie and felt your heart pound as the characters face danger? Or perhaps you've been overcome with emotion during a movie with a sad story. What you see on the screen is not real, but your emotions most definitely are. Anything that has your adrenaline pumping just before you go to bed can only disrupt your sleep. (Even if you keep the TV in a room that's more appropriate for it – your living room, for example – you should turn it off a good 45 minutes before bedtime.)

Finally, if you fall asleep while watching TV when you reach the momentary wakefulness that separates cycles of your sleep, you're far more likely to rise into consciousness – the TV's sound and the flickering lights will bring you round – especially as you'll then have to make an effort to turn off the TV. Anything that forces you to engage with reality makes it harder for you to fall back to sleep.

... *work*

I know at least half-a-dozen people who on a regular basis go to bed with an armful of papers that they need to read before the morning, or even worse with a laptop. Your bedroom is not an office. Your mind associates work with being alert, focused, driven. None of which is conducive to sleep. Furthermore, solving problems or analyzing data are active processes at a time when your brain needs to wind down.

Keeping out work also includes closing down your phone during the night, especially if you have a smartphone and could otherwise receive texts and emails at all hours. If you want to keep your phone on for emergencies, make sure it's turned to silent (including turning off the vibrate function) and in airplane mode. If you can't change your settings so that the screen doesn't light up if an email or text comes in, put your silent phone in a nearby drawer.

... *pets*

It's estimated that more than 20 percent of people who visit the Mayo Clinic Sleep Disorders Center in the USA complaining of insomnia share their bedroom with a pet. However, animals do not make good bedfellows. Their sleeping patterns do not exactly imitate ours, many dogs snore or scratch, and cats get up to stretch, prowl or pounce. Furthermore, disease can be passed easily from pets to humans through bed sharing – salmonella, parasites and plague have all occurred in people who co-sleep with cats or dogs.

If you've been used to having your dog or cat sleep with you – and if they've been used to doing it – getting them out of your bedroom may require some effort. First, put your pet out and shut your bedroom door. Cats may protest (by yowling or scratching), but can be easily distracted with a toy to play with in another room (itself shut off, if possible), or a snug cat basket put somewhere warm.

For dogs it's a simple matter of training and tough love. Buy a dog bed and put it as far away from your room as possible. If the dog starts scratching at your door, without speaking to it take it back to its own bed – and keep doing that all night if you have to. The process is rather like training a child to sleep in his or her own room. It may take a few weeks of sleepless nights, but you and the dog will get there in the end.

Bedroom ambience

The temperature, light, noise levels and your bed are all crucial factors in making your bedroom a perfect place to sleep. I'll cover all these in detail over the subsequent pages. In the meantime, also consider the colour of your sleeping space – colours that relax you and make you feel content and calm are best. Try peaceful whites, pale blues or calming greens, which studies show make it easier for us to fall asleep.

One way to help your bedroom feel calm is to cut down on the clutter. Put your clothes away in the wardrobe, drawers or laundry every night. Avoid boxes or bags of sundry items on the top of your wardrobe or under your bed. If you need to use under-bed storage, buy suitably shallow containers with lids. Keep surfaces clear – dedicate a drawer in a bedside table for toiletries or jewelry, for example.

SLEEP THERAPY

BEDROOM FENG SHUI

Feng shui (from the Chinese meaning "wind–water") is an ancient system of orientation believed to harmonize the flow of *qi* energy through our environment. The following are three of the most important feng shui considerations when laying out a bedroom:

1. Position your bed-head against a solid wall (but don't hang anything above the bed) and so that you can lie in bed and see beyond the bedroom door. In these ways you'll feel more secure. Try not to face the door, though, as some feng shui practitioners call feet pointing toward the door the "death position". If you have more than one door from your bedroom, try to position your bed so that it's not in line with any of them.
2. Make sure your mattress is raised off the floor on a bedframe and has space under and on either side of it. In Chinese terms, this allows *qi* energy to flow around and under the bed freely.
3. Have a plant in your bedroom. Nature has a calming effect on the mind and body (just looking at nature can lower blood pressure). However, don't forget to water it! An unhealthy plant creates an unhappy environment. If you're hopeless with plants, choose a picture of a natural scene, perhaps a forest, a flower or even a beautiful garden, to hang on the wall instead.

Finally, think about how you lay out your bedroom furniture. For ideas, you could try taking some tips from the Chinese art of feng shui (see box, above).

TEMPERATURE CONTROL

US President Benjamin Franklin (1706–1790) thought it was impossible to sleep when it was too hot, so he used two beds in a bedroom that he kept as cool as possible. When he got too hot in one bed, he moved to the other. He also slept in the nude. His concerns over getting his nighttime temperature just right were well founded.

Your body has to begin a process of cooling down to trigger the onset of sleep (see box, p.15). If you can't cool down, you'll find it harder to drop off. Equally, though, you're more likely to wake up at the wrong time (probably at around three or four in the morning when your body temperature is at its lowest) if you're too cold.

The key underlying message is that you'll find it easier to fall asleep if your bedroom is cool, but you're more likely to sleep through the night if you have bed linen that prevents you from getting too cold.

It's very hard to advise how to create an "ideal" bedroom temperature, as there are so many influences over how warm or cold you feel at night, not least your own unique sensitivity to heat and cold. In addition, the average room temperature in your house is probably not exactly the same as even your closest neighbour's – it will depend on such things as the heating, insulation and air-conditioning systems you have, whether or not you have double glazing and even the material your curtains are made from. What you prefer to wear to bed, the position you sleep in and whether or not you share your bed with someone else are also fundamental to how warm or cold you feel at night. All these factors, and more, influence *your* temperature in *your* bedroom in *your* home, and make it different from anyone else's.

Some years ago a hotel chain in the UK asked me what temperature they should keep the rooms at in order to keep fuel bills low, but stop guests complaining they were too cold. I told them 18°C (64.5°F) and I would stick by that as a general rule. However, other studies show that around 16°C (60°F) is better. You have to work with your own uniqueness – and if you share a room, go for the cooler of the two preferred temperatures and give your room-mate an extra blanket!

In hot weather/"I'm too hot to fall asleep"

In order to cool you down, your body will try to expel heat from the top of your head, and from your hands and your feet. You'll also sweat. If you don't fall asleep easily because generally you're too hot when you go to bed, try the following:

- Wear cotton or silk nightclothes, even in preference to sleeping naked. Natural fibres wick away moisture from your skin, which in turn allows the body's cooling mechanisms to work properly. Make sure your nightclothes are loose-fitting and comfortable. If you do prefer to sleep naked, adhere to the following point ...
- Use sheets (top and bottom), and a duvet cover if you have a duvet, made from natural fibres.
- If you can, consider sleeping with your legs spread apart rather than curling yourself up into a ball. Spreading your sleeping surface area will help to keep you cool.
- Try to circulate air through your room. If you don't have a ceiling fan or air conditioning, leave your bedroom door open. If you live in a house and sleep upstairs, leave the loft hatch open. If it's safe (and quiet) to do so, leave the windows open, too. You can also invest in a stand-alone fan – larger versions operate more quietly, if you think the noise might be an issue.
- Consider what your mattress is made from. Some people find that futon mattresses are generally cooler, because they're filled with natural fibres that wick away sweat from the body. If you don't want to invest in a new mattress, try using a mattress protector made from cotton wadding.
- For some, it can work to keep your pillow in the refrigerator during the day, taking it out just before you go to bed.
- If things are particularly bad and you're simply tossing and turning, get out of bed and, for an instant cooler, run your wrists and hands under the cold tap for a few minutes. Dry your hands and go straight back to bed.
- If your room is too hot at night during the winter because you've had the central heating on all day, I advise keeping the radiator in your bedroom turned off, day and night. If that would make spending time there during the day too cold, turn it off at least four hours before you go to bed, and leave it off all night. Follow the guidelines below for keeping warm during the night when your body temperature drops.

In cold weather/"I'm too cold to sleep well"

Even in cold weather, keeping the heating on during the night in your bedroom is often not the answer. If your room is cold, you have the best possible platform to get your nighttime temperature right. Apart from anything else, central heating will cause your sinuses to block up, which means you're likely to develop a stuffy nose that in itself might wake you. Keep warm by having bedclothes that do the job. Have you heard the old adage "snug as a bug in a rug"? That has to be you.

- Use cotton or other natural fibre bedding to ensure that you lose heat effectively as you try to drop off to sleep, but that during the night you have bedding over you to keep you warm.
- Try using layers of blankets rather than a lone duvet. That way, if you find you've overestimated you can pull a blanket off during the night (or put it back on if you're then too cold). Most of us are able to do this without rousing fully from sleep. This also works well if you share a bed with someone who doesn't share your need for extra layers!
- If you prefer to sleep with a duvet, use one that's a suitable weight for the colder months, and as long as you aren't allergic to natural fibres find one filled with feathers and down. Not only will natural fibres allow your skin to breathe during the night, they're more likely to fall snugly round you.
- Use a mattress pad so that you don't lose heat into your mattress. A blanket underneath your sheet can help, too. I don't recommend electric blankets. You mustn't keep one on overnight for safety reasons, in which case it will keep you warm at the wrong point – as you're trying to fall asleep.
- Try wearing flannel cotton nightclothes, which are warmer than the thin cotton you might use for the summer months. Make sure your nightclothes are loose-fitting, though, as you still want your skin to breathe. If you like to sleep in the nude, use flannel cotton sheets, as well as your duvet, to keep warm.
- Wear bedsocks, or in extreme circumstances even gloves or a hat to help keep in the heat. However, unless your room is cold rather than cool, this may make it harder to fall asleep.

Overall, once you've discovered what works for your body tempera-ture, stick to it. If you share a bed with a partner who has different temperature needs, you'll need to concentrate on the solutions that can work for each individual – beginning with what you each wear to bed.

INTO THE DARKNESS

From our first months of life, we develop the psychological association that darkness triggers sleep. Of course, physiological associations come into play, too. Darkness triggers the release of a host of hormones, including melatonin – the "vampire" hormone (see box, p.16) that sets our biological clock. We cease secretion of melatonin when the dawn breaks, providing one of the signals that tells the body it's time to wake up. In order to stay asleep, we need darkness so that there's no cessation (momentary or otherwise) in our melatonin secretion.

For many years, scientists thought that light had to be very bright (like sunlight) to stop melatonin secretion. Now we know that isn't true. More recent research suggests that even the light of a nightlight is enough to trick the brain into thinking that dawn is breaking.

Keep light out

One of the simplest and most effective things you can do to encourage fully restorative sleep is to make sure you have the best-quality curtains or blackout blinds you can afford. If you have curtains, make sure they're lined. Blackout-lining (available in fabric stores) is ideal.

If you have a streetlamp outside your bedroom window, you may find that the light creeps in around the edges of the curtains. Blinds are often better than curtains in these circumstances, as they tend to lie flatter against the window. Choose those that fit inside the window recess, rather than outside it. You could also try talking to your local authority about turning out the street lighting between certain hours of the night.

Finally, a word of warning. Your body does need morning light to reset your body clock for the day. If you find you're waking later in the mornings, leave a small gap in the curtains on one or two nights a week so that ambient light creeps in to keep your body clock in sync.

Don't bring light in

I once heard a friend reassure his daughter that rather than being scary, "the darkness is your friend". Unless you're very afraid of darkness (and by that I mean actually phobic), avoid using nightlights, or leaving a hall or landing light on and your bedroom door open.

If you regularly get up to go to the loo at night and you're worried about tripping, find nightlights for the passageway between your room and the loo that use red bulbs rather than white ones – and never put on the overhead light. The brain doesn't register red light as encroaching daylight, so red light doesn't interrupt melatonin secretion.

If there are no conveniently located sockets, keep a torch with a red bulb beside your bed and use that instead. Alternatively, it's now possible to buy battery-operated movement-sensitive nightlights that come on to emit a gradual and gentle glow if they detect movement during the night. You can position them strategically along corridors and in the bathroom. See the Resources on page 208 for details.

NOISE AND SLEEP

According to research by the World Health Organisation (WHO), a staggering one in five Europeans is subjected to noise that disturbs their sleep. In fact, noise disturbance is generally considered to be one of the main causes of insomnia. Interestingly, we're not born with such sensitivity to noise – babies are able to sleep through most loud noises.

In a quiet street you're likely to be woken by a sudden, unexpected noise – such as the roar of a lone car, the screech of a siren, or the bark of a dog. Noise becomes a problem only when it's persistent and it frequently disturbs your sleep, manifesting as shifts in sleeping position and increased heart rate (not necessarily coming to full wakefulness). In an attempt to address the issue of noise-related sleep disturbance, the WHO released guidelines that stipulate that, on average, no household should be subjected to noise levels greater than 40dB. This sound level is equivalent to the noise you would expect from a residential street at night. As soon as the noise levels tip consistently above 55dB (average, per night), which is the noise you would expect from a busy road with a more or less constant stream of traffic, residents run the risk of developing high blood pressure, increasing susceptibility to heart attack. To put all this into context, a normal-level conversation operates at about 60dB. These findings are based on research in Europe that was conducted over six years – such rigorous and lengthy analysis makes the results all the more troubling.

Of course, noise disturbance doesn't always have to come from outside. A clock ticking in the bedroom will keep some people awake, as will a snoring bed partner. And it's not only the *presence* of noise that can be a problem – research suggests that it takes only a week to ten days to become accustomed to sleeping with low-level noise, such as a ticking clock. If we then try to sleep in a room without that regular noise, the silence itself becomes a sleep thief. First things first, though: what can be done to reduce noise disturbance at night?

White noise

When you put together all the colours of the rainbow, you get white light. When you put together all the sound frequencies, you get white noise. People variously describe white noise as sounding like the noise of a fan, the static of an untuned radio, the whoosh of wind through trees, or the rhythmical drum of heavy rain on a window.

White noise has a neutralizing effect on other noises, and is therefore able to mask them. A simple way to look at it is to think of a single tone. If you play this tone on its own, your ears pick out the sound and your brain interprets it. If you played two tones at the same time, you could probably still pick out one tone over the other. Your brain might even be able to do that if three or four tones were played at the same time. However, if you played 20,000 tones at the same time, your brain would not be able to identify one from another, instead perceiving an indistinguishable flat hum. White noise works as a sleep aid because your brain simply adds any room noise to the mêlée of 20,000 frequencies played together.

There are many, many gadgets that you can buy or apps that you can download to your smartphone that are intended to stream white noise. Some are for playing through headphones and others are intended for

SLEEP CLINIC

My husband finds the traffic noise outside our home really disturbing for his sleep, but I sleep through it. Why?

You could be one of a lucky few. Preliminary research conducted in 2010 at Harvard University in the USA has indicated that some people may be better at blocking out noise at night than others. We already know that sleep spindles (see p.20) block sensory information passing into the areas of the brain that perceive noise. The research team revealed that those participants in their study who experienced greater numbers of sleep spindles were less likely to be roused from sleep when a telephone rang or the noise of traffic was played in the sleep laboratory. The evidence is not conclusive, but it does suggest that some of us might be genetically predisposed to finding noise much less of a problem than others.

the room at large. You'll need to discuss with your partner which you should go for, as well as considering whether or not you would find it uncomfortable to wear headphones in bed.

If you want to try this technique, I suggest opting for a white-noise gadget that doesn't loop the sound but generates sound as it goes. This is because your brain is very good at picking out the tiny skip in sound as the loop begins again, which in itself can become disturbing.

Ear plugs

Probably the simplest option for blocking out noise is to invest in a pair of earplugs. My advice is to buy the best ear plugs you can afford.

Ear plugs can reduce sound by up to 30dB, so can be extremely effective, but only if they fit properly. Find a pair that completely blocks your ear canal (the part of your ear that carries sound to your eardrum). Experiment with different shapes and sizes, or ideally look for brands that mould to the shape of your ear. You could even try talking to your doctor about investing in a pair that's custom-made.

SLEEP CLINIC

I'm worried that if I try to block out sound so that I sleep better, I won't hear my children call for me in the night.

There's no doubt that the main problem with anything that blocks sound (whether that's because it's become part of white noise or because you're wearing ear plugs) is that you run the risk of not hearing something you need to hear – such as your baby crying, or a smoke alarm. Ear plugs are particularly effective at blocking out low tones (such as the hum of traffic), and less good at stopping high-pitched sounds, which means you're still likely to hear the urgent screech of an alarm or your children's cries. In fact, women in particular have a primal instinct to hear their children, and even white noise is unlikely to drown them out. Nonetheless, if you don't want to risk blocking out sound altogether, try the alternative solutions below. These leave your hearing unmuffled, but should help to reduce the impact of noise on your sleep.

Foam ear plugs tend to be more effective, but silicone ones may be more comfortable.

When you fit the earplug, twist it so that it's as small as it will go before placing it inside your ear. This way it will expand within your ear canal, filling the cavity as much as possible. The downside of earplugs is that you may become more susceptible to ear infections if you regularly block up your ears.

Other solutions to noise disturbance

Finally, the following pointers will help to reduce noise disturbance, but without muffling your hearing.

- Use heavy curtains in your bedroom, which will not only block out light (see p.49) but also reduce noise.
- Keep your windows closed at night and use a quiet fan or air-conditioner to circulate air in hot weather.

- If you don't already have it, consider double or triple glazing or even secondary glazing for your bedroom.
- If snoring is the problem, ask your partner to read pages 170–171 and follow the advice to try to solve the problem.

MAKING YOUR BED

If the real princess in the Hans Christian Andersen fairytale *The Princess and the Pea* could feel the pea beneath twenty mattresses and twenty feather beds, she really needed to examine her sensitivity to her sleeping surface! Nonetheless, she couldn't get a proper night's sleep. In my opinion your bed, and more specifically your mattress, is the single most important component of your sleeping environment.

Size matters

Sleep Council guidelines in the UK recommend that your mattress is between 10cm and 15cm (4 and 6in) longer than the tallest person who sleeps on it. It's unlikely that you'll sleep with your head perfectly aligned to one end of the mattress, so having a bit of extra length enables you to move around, including shuffling up and down, during the night without your feet dangling off the end.

In practice this means that if you're 182cm (6ft) tall, your mattress should be 192 to 197cm (6ft 4in to 6ft 6in) long. The approximate length for a regular single or double mattress is 190cm (6ft 3in), whereas kingsize and superking tend to be around 200cm (6ft 6in) long. If you or your partner is over 190cm tall, you may need to consider having a mattress (and a bedframe) specially made for you.

If you're sharing a bed with a partner, your mattress needs to be wide enough to give you both space to move around without disturbing the other. Choose a new mattress together. Lie side by side on your backs and put your hands behind your head, elbows out to the sides. If the bed is wide enough, neither of you should have your outermost elbow hanging off the side; and your innermost elbows shouldn't touch.

If you sleep alone in a single bed, make sure that it's wide enough for you to roll over fully in both directions without feeling that you're

SLEEP THERAPY

TESTING YOUR MATTRESS

Use these steps to assess the suitability of your present mattress and any mattress you consider buying in the future.

1. Lie in your normal sleeping position. Do you feel supported where you need support and comfort everywhere else? If there are pressure points on your body, the mattress is too firm. If you feel that you're sinking into the mattress, it's too soft.
2. Turn over onto your side and roll back again to the other side. You should be able to turn easily from side to side. If that's the case, your spine is horizontal and your body properly supported, and you're far less likely to wake up when you shuffle about in your sleep. If rolling takes effort, the mattress is too soft.
3. Lie on one side. Put your hand between the mattress and the natural indent at your waist. You should be able to slide your hand under with a snug fit. If you have to squeeze your hand through with effort, the mattress is too soft. If the gap makes it very easy to get your hand through, the mattress is too hard.

going to roll off. Ideally, choose the widest single bed you can for the space available; or if you have the space and budget, sleep in a double.

Soft or hard?

First, let's imagine that even if you have a partner this bed is just for you. The firmness of your mattress depends on a number of things, beginning with your weight. The heavier you are, the more you're going to sink into a mattress, so the firmer it will need to be to give you adequate support. Spend a few moments testing your mattress now, using the experiment in the box on the following page.

When you buy a new mattress you must test it properly before you commit – and you can't do that by lying on it momentarily in one position in the showroom. Run through all the tests in the box on the following page *and* spend at least ten minutes lying on it in your normal sleeping position. Don't be shy: ten minutes is only a fraction of the time you'll actually spend sleeping on that mattress if you buy it, so it's the least you owe your sleeping health. Finally, there are no industry standards for mattress firmness – what's firm in one brand may be considered medium in another, and so on. Always test a new mattress before you buy and don't rely on what you had before.

Once you've found your perfect mattress, you need to see if it matches your partner's preferences, too. If it does, life is easy. If, however, you have different needs – and particularly if there's a difference of 20kg (42lb) in your weights – you might consider buying two single mattresses, one to accommodate each of you, that zip together. The type of mattress filling you buy can also help to make sleep more comfortable for both of you, and I cover that next.

Not all mattresses are created equal

There are two main types of mattress: foam and sprung. If you're going for a foam mattress, I recommend memory foam (technically called temperature-sensitive visco-elastic). This was first used to cushion astronauts' bodies as they re-entered our atmosphere. Memory foam mattresses respond to the body's heat, moulding to the contour of your shape and remoulding as you move. Their aim is to make sure that your body is always supported and your spine is straight. They have the added benefit of being an inhospitable environment for dust mites and bed bugs, making them a great choice if you suffer from allergies.

Sprung mattresses are made from large metal coils and they come in three main types:

- Open spring (or open coil) mattresses are made up of rows of individual coil springs linked together and held in position by a border wire. Better-quality versions have a thick mattress wadding over the top so that you can't feel the springs. However, compared with other types of mattress coil, open springs are more likely to shift within the structure, which means the mattress can become uneven and uncomfortable.
- Continuous spring mattresses are made from a single piece

SLEEP CLINIC

My daughter suffers from asthma and her laboured breathing disturbs her sleep. How can I keep her mattress dust-mite-free?

Asthma and allergies can be brought on by allergens found on the faeces of house dust mites. The simplest way to prevent dust mites from living in a mattress is to buy a mattress made of foam (see main text, opposite). However, in sprung mattresses using protective covers, and regular airing and vacuum-cleaning can slow down mite infestation, although it won't prevent it altogether. Mites live by drinking the water naturally present in the air (humidity). Another way to keep them at bay is to invest in a dehumidifier. When the average daily indoor humidity is lower than 50 percent, mites can't survive, and within several months the mite population can be dramatically reduced or even culled altogether.

of wire that is coiled up and down and knitted together. The tighter the coil, the firmer the mattress will be. The benefit of this type of mattress is that there are no individual springs to move out of place and cause obvious lumps in the bed.

• Pocket-spring mattresses contain lots of sewn-together fabric pockets, each housing a single spring. The more pockets (more springs) you have – some have several thousand – the better quality the mattress as there are more places where the mattress will "give" to the contours of your body. If you're sharing your bed with someone else, more pockets means that the mattress will give more independently for each of you.

A word of warning when choosing your new mattress – treat sceptically any claims that particular brands are orthopaedically or medically proven to reduce back pain or stiffness. So much depends on the individual – body shape, weight, sleeping position, and so on – that there is no one-size-fits-all option. Shop with an open mind and don't be influenced by manufacturers' claims of medical supremacy.

Take a turn

Should you turn your mattress? Not if you have a memory-foam mattress, but sprung mattresses do need the odd spin. When you first get a new mattress, spin it top to bottom (rather than turning it over, end over end) once a week for the first three or four weeks, and then once every two months thereafter. Many modern mattresses don't need an end-over-end turn at all, but check your manufacturer's recommendations. If you do need to flip the mattress, ask someone to help you.

Other bed basics

Your mattress isn't the only component of your bed. The frame, pillows and bedding can also affect your chances of a good night's sleep.

- Your bed frame influences how soft or firm a mattress feels. If you have a bedstead or divan with a mesh or sprung base (rather than a solid or slatted base), the mattress will feel softer. Bear this in mind if you buy one without the other.
- Choose your pillow carefully. As you lie down on your back or side, your head and neck should naturally align with your spine. This way you'll avoid putting stress on your neck and waking with pain (your head is the heaviest part of your body, so it needs good support). Feather pillows keep their shape for longer than manmade-fibre pillows; although manmade fibres are a good choice for allergy sufferers. Memory foam pillows mould to your posture and don't harbour mites and bed bugs.
- Sprung mattress toppers or protectors help save your mattress from sweat, which can attract mites and bugs. They're also easy to wash to keep your bed hygiene at good levels.
- Smooth, clean sheets are more conducive to restful sleep. Use a fitted cotton bottom sheet, which is breathable and also less likely to wrinkle beneath you. Tuck in your cotton topsheet properly at the end of your bed, and particularly on the bottom corners (think "hospital corners"), so that it doesn't become

SLEEP CLINIC

I've had my mattress for seven years. Does a mattress have a shelf life and should I buy a new one?

The Furniture Industry Research Association in the UK has shown that a mattress can deteriorate by as much as 70 percent over ten years. Most sleep experts recommend ten years as being the trigger point for a new investment. However, if you answer yes to any of the following questions, regardless of how long you've had your current mattress, it might be time to go shopping.

1. Do you wake up with stiffness, aches or pains (especially in your shoulders, neck, back or hips) that ease as the day progresses?
2. Do you remember when you slept better on your present mattress – perhaps six months or a year ago?
3. Does your mattress show signs of visible wear and tear (frayed edges, springs that protrude, loose or broken stitching)?
4. Can you see any obvious dips or sagging in the mattress?

tangled as you move in your sleep. Wash your bed linen at least once a week, and your duvet once a month. (See also pages 45–9 for advice about temperature and your choice of linen.)

RITUALS FOR SLEEP

Good sleep hygiene includes two "ritual" components: the way in which you schedule your sleep and the activities you undertake in order to prepare your body for sleep.

Good sleep–wake habits

One of the most important things you can do to get a proper night's sleep and to wake feeling refreshed in the morning is to have a regular bedtime and to get up at the same time every day – even on the days when you have no pressing appointment to get up for. Your body likes routine. If you're having trouble sleeping you need to condition it to feel sleepy at the right time at night and to wake up so that you feel alert at the right time in the morning. Take a look at the box opposite and follow its advice to set your sleep–wake cycle.

Of course, there will be times when you go to bed later than your usual bedtime. As long as you've conditioned your body successfully into a healthy sleep–wake cycle, the occasional late night isn't going to upset all your hard work. However, even if you go to bed later than is typical, get up at your normal waking time. Your body will recover the sleep debt by maxing out your deep sleep the following night – but if you sleep in, you run the risk of not feeling sleepy at your usual bedtime. If you absolutely need to grab some extra shut-eye long before bedtime, take a nap in the early afternoon and set your alarm to wake you after 30 minutes. Then, go to bed at your normal time.

A word about naps: they should be the exceptions rather than the rule – only when you really need to make up for a very late night and only occasionally. Many nighttime insomnia sufferers reveal themselves to be daytime nappers. In most cases, napping is a sleep thief.

Bedtime rituals

If you've set up your sleep–wake cycle, you'll be going to bed at a time when you feel naturally sleepy. Nonetheless, a bedtime ritual helps to reinforce the message to your brain that it's time to sleep. Your ritual doesn't have to be elaborate or even very long, but it must be calming. For example, you could:

• turn off the TV an hour before your bedtime and do something
  quiet and contemplative, perhaps along with a warm glass of
  milk or a soporific herbal tea (see p.201)

then

• lock the front and back doors, and turn out the lights except
  the light in your bathroom and a low-wattage bedside lamp

then

• get into your nightclothes and wash your face and brush your
  teeth, turning out the bathroom light as you leave the room

SLEEP THERAPY

SETTING YOUR SLEEP–WAKE CYCLE

The following might affect your social life, but shouldn't affect your working or school life at all. For simplicity, I've assumed that you want to condition your body so that it's ready for sleep at 11pm and ready to wake up at 7am. If these times don't suit you (for example, if 10pm until 6am works better with your schedule), that's fine – you can change the times, but try to make sure they allow for seven to eight hours of shut-eye every night.

1. You'll need to set aside four weeks for this, because conditioning your body into a new routine won't happen overnight (excuse the pun). Clear your diary of all social engagements that would keep you out late in the evening and let your friends and family know that you are not contactable between 11pm and 7am.
2. Set your alarm clock for 7am and make sure that it's on its loudest setting so that it wakes you straightaway. Put the alarm clock out of reach so you have to get out of bed to stop its noise.
3. On the first night of your new routine, practise your pre-sleep rituals in time for you to be actually in your bed by 11pm with your eyes closed, regardless of whether or not you feel sleepy.
4. When your alarm goes off, get up. Immediately. Go to the window, open the curtains and let light flood in. If it's still dark outside, turn on all the lights. Artificial light isn't as effective at setting your biological clock as natural light, but it's better than trying to wake up in the gloom.
5. Repeat this ritual every night and morning for the whole four weeks, by the end of which you should have reconditioned your body into a healthy sleep–wake cycle. You'll know you've done it because you'll naturally feel sleepy at 11pm and you'll be on the cusp of wakefulness when the alarm sounds in the morning.

then
- sit or lie on a folded blanket on your bedroom floor and practise a ten-minute muscle relaxation (see box, opposite) or the breathing relaxation on page 71

then
- slide under the covers and turn out the bedside lamp

Some people include a warm bath in their bedtime rituals – but anything from putting out the cat to luxuriating in an aromatherapy bubble bath can form part of the routine as long as you practise it in the same sequence and with regularity. Avoid anything that might stimulate your body at this time – television, work, vigorous exercise, or conversations with your partner about children, the house, money, or other emotive issues do not make for a successful bedtime ritual. Look at the advice for stress-free slumber on page 70, too.

See the light

It may seem like a long way until your next bedtime, but the first hour of your waking is an important time for setting your biological clock. Dawning light filters through your eyelids and will begin to rouse you from sleep up to two hours before you actually wake up. This is one way in which light helps to set the biological clock so that it's in tune with the Earth's 24-hour cycle of light and dark. But there's another way, too. In the sleep hygiene review (see pp.38–41), I asked if you ever make a point of getting the daylight on your face when you wake up. Making this part of your waking ritual will help to prepare your body for its next night of sleep.

Facing daylight first thing doesn't mean sitting in the garden or on the terrace for an hour, come rain or shine, with your morning coffee. It's much easier and quicker than that. All you have to do is to open the window and let the light flood your face for a few moments. You could even leave the windows closed if it's too cold or wet to open them. The light receptors in your retinas (see p.14) send chemical messages to your brain to confirm that the morning is here and that it's time to wake up. If your biological clock is set to give you a wake-up call at

SLEEP THERAPY

RELAXING YOUR MUSCLES

Progressive muscle relaxation releases tension from all the body's muscle groups in turn. Lie on your bedroom floor on a yoga mat if you have one, or otherwise on a folded blanket.

1. Lie on your back, arms by your sides and your legs straight, but not rigid. Allow your knees and toes to fall naturally outward.
2. Focus your attention on the top of your head. Screw up your brow into a deep frown. Hold it tight, then release it.
3. Scrunch your shoulders up toward your ears. Hold for a few seconds, then release. Feel your shoulders sink into the floor beneath you, and your neck lengthen again naturally.
4. Scrunch up your arms and chest by pulling your hands into fists, folding your arms at the elbows and tucking your fists under your chin. Hold, then release – first your chest, then the tops of your arms, then your lower arms (unfolding them to your sides again) and finally your fists.
5. Tense your buttocks. Hold them tight, then let them go so that they sink back down.
6. Pull your thigh muscles tight by locking your knees and tensing. Hold, and release allowing your hips and thighs to relax.
7. Push your heels downwards and point your toes toward the ceiling, pulling on your calf muscles and stretching the muscles in the souls of your feet. Hold and release.
8. Curl up your toes tightly. When you release them, feel the tingle as the tension dissipates.
9. Lie still for a few minutes and give your body an internal self-check. Can you feel any areas of tension that you haven't released? If so, consciously tense the muscles in that area and then let go so that the tension ebbs away, too. When you're ready, get into bed. Your body is ready for sleep.

the correct time in the morning, its natural rhythm will help to prepare you to feel sleepy at the right time in the evening, too.

THE LIFESTYLE FACTOR

From what and when we eat to how much alcohol we drink, how much stress we're under and when we exercise, all sorts of lifestyle factors impact our ability to sleep soundly. This section looks at how you can top off all the other aspects of your sleep hygiene in order to have a healthy, fulfilling lifestyle that also provides refreshing, restorative sleep.

Your weight

The purpose of this book is not to tell you that you need to reach a target weight nor what you need to eat in order to optimize your nutritional intake. However, it's important to say that being overweight is detrimental to good-quality sleep.

Many studies show that there is a connection between achieving too little sleep and gaining weight, and unfortunately it's also true that the more weight you gain, the poorer your sleep. Being overweight interferes with your breathing, because it makes it harder for your throat to stay open as it relaxes between each breath. This is why overweight people tend to snore (see pp.170–71). Being overweight also makes it harder to get comfortable in bed.

When being overweight turns into being obese, you may risk developing "sleep apnoea", which causes a momentary cessation in breathing during sleep and puts a strain on your heart. As soon as your brain realizes that it's being starved of oxygen, it wakes you up so that your breathing kicks in again. See pages 171–4 for more on this.

Overall, the message is clear: if you're overweight, try to bring your weight back to within the healthy range for your build. A combination of a nutritious diet and the right amount of physical exercise so that you burn more calories than you put in is as complex as any weight-loss programme needs to get. The important thing is to lose the weight in a way that makes your target weight sustainable into the future.

Mealtimes

The timing of your meals is one way in which your body clock aligns itself with the cycle of day and night. For this reason it's important to follow a regular mealtime schedule, with breakfast, lunch and supper at more or less the same times each day.

We also already know that it's perfectly normal to feel sleepy after a big meal, when your tummy is full (see box, p.35). For this reason, we might expect that having the day's largest meal in the evening will help the body get ready for sleep. However, it's not as simple as that.

Eating is the way in which your body derives energy. After a meal, and after any initial feelings of sluggishness have passed, you should feel refuelled and energized. Obviously, this is exactly the opposite to how you want to feel before you go to bed. The best way to eat for optimum sleep is to eat little and often. Three light but well-balanced meals a day help to prevent the energy dips of mid-afternoon, but also avoid you feeling overfull or overenergized when you go to bed.

The kinds of food you eat at supper time are also important. As the 17th-century British aristocrat Lord Chesterfield once said, "A light supper, a good night's sleep, and a fine morning have often made a hero of the same man who, by indigestion, a restless night, and a rainy morning would have proved a coward." Certainly, indigestion and heartburn are often cited as reasons for preventing sleep. If you're prone to either of these, try keeping a food diary, noting down everything you eat and drink, and see if you can establish which foods cause the problem. Once you know, eliminate them from your diet – or at the very least from your evening meal.

Generally, though, a healthy diet that features a range of fresh foods, including plenty of fruits and vegetables and dietary fibre, is good for the quality of your sleep. High-sugar, high-fat foods are harder for your body to digest, which means that they are much more likely to keep you awake as your gut tries to move them through your system.

One important rule of thumb for everyone is to eat at least three to four hours before you retire for the night. This way, your body has time to digest your food before you try to go to sleep.

SLEEP CLINIC
___

My husband tells me that I should eat lettuce at bedtime to help me get to sleep. Can this really be true?

The simple answer is no, unless you want to eat it in such large quantities that it would probably give you a terribly bad stomach that keeps you awake anyway. Lettuce does contain tiny traces of two chemicals – lactucarium and hyoscyamine – that do have a soporific effect on the body. However, the amounts in lettuce are so small that you would need to eat a lot of it (and ideally on its own) for them to have any effect. You'd be better to ensure that you're getting good levels of calcium (in dairy products, as well as broccoli and spinach) in your diet, which the body uses in the manufacture of melatonin. Equally, magnesium deficiency has been linked with insomnia, so make sure you're getting plenty of this mineral, too. You can find it in dark green leafy vegetables, as well as bananas and dried apricots. Overall, a warm cup of milk at bedtime is likely to be of far more help to you than a bowl of lettuce.

Alcohol

Although alcohol is in theory a sedative, its soporific effects hold true only if it is drunk in moderation. More than a glass of wine shortly before bedtime has the opposite effect. This is primarily because alcohol is dehydrating and diuretic: while you might fall asleep easily, you're likely to wake in the night feeling thirsty and needing the loo.

More worryingly, research in the USA in the 1980s showed that alcohol consumption can lower levels of oxygen in the blood and increase susceptibility to sleep apnoea (see pp.171–4). Oxygen levels remained lower than "normal" not only on the night after the drinking occurred, but on the following night, too. More recently, in 2011, researchers studied the relationship between alcohol and the stages of sleep. They discovered that although alcohol may induce sleep initially, overall there were fewer periods of deep and dreaming sleep during the night, and that in the morning study participants generally reported feeling as though they hadn't slept at all. Indeed, many alcoholics say that they are also insomniacs, supporting the theory that alcohol interferes with the restorative powers of sleep.

We're all different, and alcohol tolerance levels vary from person to person. You can be really sure whether or not alcohol has a consistently negative effect on your sleep only by becoming teetotal for, say, six weeks, and then reintroducing an evening alcoholic drink and monitoring its effects on the quality of your sleep. You may find that a single drink, or two drinks, once or twice a week a few hours before bedtime has very little effect on your sleep quality – or you may find that your good night's sleep relies upon total abstention.

The problem with stimulants

I'm not someone who demands that their clients never let another cup of coffee pass their lips. In fact, I think a cup of coffee as a morning pick-me-up can be a good idea. Nevertheless, the simple fact is that if you want to improve the quality of your sleep, you need to steer clear of caffeine after lunchtime every day. Caffeine is found in coffee, black tea, green tea, carbonated drinks and energy drinks, and in all cocoa products, from hot chocolate drinks to bars of chocolate.

The stimulant effects of caffeine can take effect in only 15 minutes, and it can take several hours for your body to eliminate the caffeine fully. The older you are, the longer its effects are active, but on average caffeine metabolization takes between three and six hours. Caffeine disrupts your body's use of the neuromodulator adenosine to promote drowsiness. Specific receptors in the brain perceive the caffeine molecules and think that they're adenosine. Instead of latching on to adenosine (making you drowsy), the receptors hook up with the caffeine. The adenosine sleep-promoting signals then can't get through, so the wakefulness-promoting parts of the brain remain active.

Interestingly, in 2012 research students at Stanford University in the USA experimented to see if larks or owls were more susceptible to the effects of caffeine in relation to the quality of their sleep. They discovered that the owls (those who like to stay up late at night; see box,

SLEEP SCIENCE

AMPHETAMINES

Amphetamines (or *alpha-methylphenethylamines* to give them their full name) are drugs that primarily promote wakefulness, reduce fatigue and can induce feelings of euphoria and sociability. They may also be prescribed to treat narcolepsy – a condition that causes its sufferer to fall asleep at inappropriate times (see pp.154–7). However, in their illegal, "recreational" form, they appear on the market as speed, crystal meth, uppers, whiz and so on.

Apart from the fact that the law strictly prohibits the use of amphetamines outside clinical practice, these drugs have absolutely no place in the life of someone who is trying to improve the quality of their sleep. They increase heart and breathing rate, alertness and restlessness. Long-term use not only leads to insomnia, but possibly to permanent damage of the brain's cells.

p.17) in their group were far less likely to suffer the stimulant effects of caffeine during their sleeping hours than were the larks. However, the trial was conducted only on students, who tend to anyway have erratic sleeping patterns. We'd need a more representative cross-section of the population to claim for certain that the discoveries are true.

If you do need to cut down on your caffeine intake, do so gradually, reducing the number of cups you have each day by one until your intake is no longer affecting your sleep. Going "cold turkey" (stopping suddenly) can cause withdrawal symptoms – including insomnia.

Other stimulants

Caffeine is not the only stimulant in common circulation. It's estimated that around 20 percent of adult Americans smoke tobacco. The nicotine in tobacco is a powerful stimulant with an effect similar to alcohol: it reduces the amount of restorative deep sleep we get during the night. Deep sleep, REM sleep and overall sleep time are all reduced in regular smokers. This is not least because after several hours the brain starts craving nicotine to feed its addiction.

Also, rather like alcohol, nicotine increases susceptibility to sleep apnoea, with some reports claiming that smokers are three times more likely to suffer this condition than non-smokers. If you're a smoker and you think you have poor-quality sleep, you should do your utmost to quit. Although quitting might hamper your sleep initially (because of the withdrawal symptoms), persevere because in the long term your sleep quality (and other aspects of your health) will certainly improve.

Stress and relaxation

The more stressed you are and the greater the number of worries you go to bed with, the poorer the quality of your sleep. Easing the physical effects of stress and quietening anxiety are essential to a restful night.

During times of stress, a sharp rise in adrenaline pumps your muscles full of energy to prepare you to fight or flee from danger. In times gone by, you would use up this energy doing just that. Today, your body releases adrenaline when it perceives threat in just the same way – but the threat tends to require far less physical action. You wouldn't, for example, get physical when your boss tells you at 5pm one afternoon that she needs you to prepare a 30-minute presentation for the Board by 9am the following morning. In the modern world, stress tends to be more psychological – time management, the pressure of organizing an event, a vacation, a family, and so on. With emotional and mental stress, adrenaline doesn't get burned off. Instead, it's stored as muscle tension, which is as bad news for your sleep as the mental chatter.

There are many excellent books available on stress relief. As far as your sleep is concerned, they tend to offer two important messages:
- Every day set aside time to let go of as much of your daytime stress as possible, so that you can go to sleep with a quiet mind. Even if you can't be worry-free, aim to press the pause button on your anxiety. Take a look at the box on the following page for some ideas that you can work into your bedtime routine to help you shelve your worries overnight.
- Try to do something physical every day to release some pent-up

SLEEP THERAPY
_____

YOUR TIMETABLE FOR STRESS-FREE SLEEP

Try implementing the following tips every evening, so that you
can go to bed without carrying your worries with you. If you like,
you can make them a part of your bedtime routine (see pp.60–2).

During the evening:
1. Make a list of any meetings or engagements you have tomorrow
   and prepare everything you need – from your keys and wallet to
   any documentation or papers you need for the day.
2. Prepare your clothes for tomorrow, as well as your packed lunch
   or other necessities. If you have school-age children, prepare their
   school clothes, lunches and bags, too.

One to two hours before you intend to go to bed:
1. Make a list of any items that you meant to do today, but didn't
   get round to. These will be your top priorities for tomorrow.
   Then, add anything else that you'd like to achieve if you have
   time. Put the list in your work bag and clear it from your mind.
2. Turn off your TV and do something calming. Don't begin any
   contentious discussions with other household members!

30 minutes before you intend to go to bed:
1. Spend ten minutes doing a quiet breathing relaxation. For
   example, you could try the yoga Humming Bee Breath exercise
   in the box opposite. Or, you could make your body the focus of
   your relaxation (see box, p.63).

adrenaline and free the tension in your muscles. A 15-minute
brisk walk, a short cycle ride, ten minutes using a skipping rope
in the garden, or ten minutes spent gently stretching are all you
need to get the adrenaline out. Do whatever suits you and your
lifestyle, but do it daily. (See over.)

SLEEP THERAPY

HUMMING BEE BREATH

This yoga breathing meditation helps to fully absorb the mind in the act of breathing and in the vibrations of the hum as it resonates through your body. It helps to relieve tension and stress, and to generate an all-pervading sense of calm.

1. Sit in a comfortable position on the floor. Rest your hands loosely in your lap. Close your eyes, drop your shoulders and become aware of your breath.
2. Relax your jaw, but keep your mouth gently closed. Breathe in through your nose as deeply as is comfortable, bearing in mind that your abdomen should rise on each inbreath, not your chest.
3. Breathe out gently through your mouth, but with your lips together so that you can make a humming sound as you do so. Try to keep the hum going for the duration of the outbreath. You can choose whatever pitch feels most comfortable and relaxing for you. During the outbreath, notice how the hum vibrates in your chest. Focus fully on this vibration.
4. Breathe in again and repeat the hum on the outbreath. Do this for six full breaths. Then, sit quietly for a few moments. Tell yourself "I am ready for sleep", then get up slowly and go to bed.

Self-fulfilling stress

I often meet people who can't sleep because they tell themselves they can't sleep. It's often that several months or even years beforehand they suffered a stressful period in their lives that resulted in insomnia. Although they may have in all other ways moved on from what happened, the insomnia remains. Then, they've become so stressed at being unable to sleep, sleep has slipped further from their grasp.

I recommend a system called autogenic training to deal with this problem. Rather like progressive muscle relaxation (see box, p.63),

SLEEP CLINIC

I've never been to a gym or for a run; exercise fills me with dread. How much do I need to do to sleep better?

If you're otherwise healthy, aim for three 30-minute exercise sessions a week doing an activity that raises your heart rate so that you feel a little breathless. If running isn't for you, try swimming, cycling or power walking. Improving your circulation, your breathing and your overall fitness will in turn improve your sleep.

However, if you suffer from stress (or if you *also* suffer from stress), and you feel uncomfortable and restless when you lie in bed, it's possible that adrenaline has built up in your muscles and you need to set it free. In this case, try just a ten-minute burst of physical activity every day (such as a ten-minute power walk), as well as an exercise to relieve muscle tension (see p.63).

you take parts of your body in turn, but this time repeat in your head a calming phrase, such as "My head feels heavy; my head feels heavy and warm; my head is resting." From your head, you move to left arm, left hand, right arm, right hand, chest, abdomen, left leg, left foot, right leg, right foot – each time repeating the phrase with the appropriate body part. To finish, repeat three times "I'm ready for sleep."

In time, your mindset should shift from one of "I can't sleep!" to "I'm ready for sleep" – and sleep should follow. How long it takes for the shift to happen will be unique to you (allow four weeks), but the positive self-talk will work once you've broken the habit of negativity.

Fit for sleep

As I've already said, exercising to release pent-up energy every day is an important form of stress relief that aids sleep. However, there may be other benefits to exercise, too. Historically, scientists have claimed that exercise improves sleep for a number of reasons. First, it tires out the muscles, which means they are primed for a period of rest. Second, exercise breaks down muscle tissue, so the body wants to induce sleep (a time of growth and restoration) to build muscle back up again. Certainly, research in Minneapolis, USA, in 2011 showed that people who exercise regularly sleep longer at night and enjoy more deep, restorative sleep (and slightly less dreaming sleep). It also found that daytime energy levels were better and that participants were able to concentrate for longer periods. Most importantly, regular exercise of a brisk walk and a little weight training reduced the incidence of sleep apnoea by 25 percent, even if the participants didn't also lose weight.

A year earlier, in 2010, researchers in Switzerland also found that exercise could improve sleep, but only if participants *believed* they were doing enough. Participants in the study who exercised frequently and were physically very fit, but who felt they needed to do more, slept more fitfully than those who did only moderate amounts of exercise but felt good about themselves and *believed* themselves to be fit.

Either way, it seems that whether it's for psychological reasons (because it makes you feel good about yourself) or physiological reasons, regular exercise is an important activity for improving your sleep. However, that's only if you engage in it at the right times of day. Exercise increases your body temperature and your metabolism, both of which are stimulating, so you need to leave at least four hours between any burst of exercise and your bedtime.

CHAPTER 4

SLEEP, AGEING AND GENDER

Why do we say that if we've had a good night's sleep we've "slept like a baby"? What is it about women that makes them more prone to complain about the quality of their sleep? And why is it that men are more often accused of snoring? Although we all sleep, the nature of our sleep changes over the course of our lives and shows different, traceable characteristics according to our gender. In this chapter I'll answer not only the questions above, but also look at the sleep of teens and adolescents and of the older generation. I'll reveal what it is about menstruation, pregnancy and menopause that can affect a woman's sleep, as well as how a man's sleep is affected by his levels of testosterone. And I'll offer guidance on how to work with your age and gender traits to help you to achieve the best-quality sleep possible.

SLEEPING BABIES, RESTED CHILDREN

During the early months after birth, a baby's rate of learning is faster than at any other time in his or her life. This means that babies need a lot of time to process new information: they need a lot of sleep.

Baby sleep is "polyphasic" – that is, babies don't have a single, long period of sleep as adults do. Rather, their sleep is broken up into several distinct periods over the course of 24 hours. Once they reach two to three months of age, most babies will take their longest sleep during the night (still waking for feeds, but going straight back to sleep again). However, it's also normal for babies to take up to a year to get the hang of sleeping through the night. By their first birthdays, though, most babies are sleeping between nine and 14 hours at night, with one long nap of between one and three hours immediately after lunch. (It's important to emphasize that there are no rights or wrongs in the early stages and what works for one tiny baby may not work for another.)

A baby's sleep cycle is not 90 minutes, but 45 to 60 minutes, gradually extending to the full 90 minutes by the time the child is about four years old. Also, unlike an adult's, a newborn's sleep is made up of only two sleep phases – non-REM and REM. Each sleep cycle is divided roughly evenly between the two phases at first. Then, periods of REM gradually reduce and non-REM gradually increase, until all the sleep phases kick in along with the 90-minute sleep cycle at around four.

Establishing good sleep health

In the first few weeks and months of a baby's life, there's no question that a baby's sleeping pattern can seem erratic, even untraceable. My advice is that once your baby reaches six to eight weeks of age you try introducing some early principles of "nighttime" behaviour.

- Implement an evening pre-sleep routine – for example, give your baby a warm bath and then dry and dress him or her in a dimly lit room before settling down to the bedtime feed. Aim for the routine to be well established (even if it's not yet fully effective) by 12 weeks.
- Avoid stimulating activities in the last hour or so before bedtime and make an effort to talk more quietly. You could even spend some time softly singing your favourite lullabies. Your baby will soon come to associate them with sleep time.
- Try not to allow your baby to fall asleep while feeding – put the baby on his or her back into the cot or crib while drowsy but still awake. (This is important for establishing a pattern of self-soothing. If the baby is used to dropping off to sleep in bed, rather than in your arms, he or she will be able to soothe

him- or herself back to sleep following a momentary period of wakefulness during the night – instead of crying out for you.)
• Remember that tiny babies do not cry to be manipulative – they cry because they need something (food, love, a nappy change or, indeed, sleep itself). If your baby wakes during the night, keep the lights off (or very low) and avoid talking. Soothe with gentle caresses and put the baby back to bed.

As your baby grows into a toddler and then a pre-schooler, you can add layers to your bedtime routine – a story, for example, for the toddler and tooth-brushing for the pre-schooler, or saying good night to a special teddy. As long as the routine is the same every night, your child will soon make the association that this pattern of behaviour is the preamble for going to sleep.

Childhood sleep problems

It's perfectly normal for children to experience some degree of sleep problem during the first years of their lives – for example, approximately 30 percent of families will have a problem with a baby crying during the night. Common childhood sleep problems include difficulty going to sleep and frequent nighttime waking. Problems are formally categorized in the International Classification of Sleep Disorders as Behavioural Insomnia of Childhood (see box, pp.78–9).

Interestingly, most of these sleep problems in infants and pre-school children do not have a physical origin, but are behaviourally based: they result from poor sleep habits or training.

Prolonged poor sleep quality, or disrupted sleep–wake schedules, can impair a child's short- and long-term memory, attention span, academic performance and ability to undertake complex tasks. Recent studies show that children with reduced sleep duration are more likely to be overweight or obese and have problems regulating their insulin and glucose levels (the precursor to metabolic syndrome, which can in turn lead to Type II diabetes). Children who sleep for fewer than ten hours a night may have an increased risk of injury than longer sleepers – probably because a child's balance, agility and co-ordination suffer

SLEEP CLINIC

Should I let my new baby sleep in my bedroom and, if so, should she be in my bed?

Overwhelming evidence suggests that having your baby in your room until he or she is six months old reduces the incidence of SIDS ("cot death") by up to 50 percent. No one knows for sure why this is so, but it might simply be that we are more attuned to our baby's breathing rhythm (and so notice if there is a pause in it) and murmurings if he or she is nearby. As a result, I strongly advise keeping your baby in your room with you for the first six months.

Keeping your baby in your own bed is called "co-sleeping". There's a great deal of controversy over whether or not this is suitable and safe for the baby. The pros are that it's much easier if you're breastfeeding to have your baby in bed with you, and some believe that babies who co-sleep grow up feeling more independent and secure. For the cons: if you're a particularly deep sleeper, you or your partner smoke (or you smoked during pregnancy), you're taking any medication, or you've drunk any alcohol before bedtime, there may be an increased risk of rolling on top of the baby, putting her at risk. My advice is that you consider all the evidence for both sides and make a decision that best suits you and your family. If you're still unsure what's best, you could invest in a cot that has a drop-down side, enabling you to put the baby up against your bed accessibly, but still in her own safe space.

when he or she is tired. Finally, a child who has not had enough sleep will be more aggressive, irritable and emotionally fragile. Over time, too little sleep may even result in clinical behavioural problems (such as hyperactivity disorder). None of this is all that surprising, of course, because these responses to lack of sleep are on a par with those we would expect for adults who clock up too few hours of slumber.

CLASSIFICATION OF CHILDHOOD SLEEP DISORDERS

The American Academy of Sleep Medicine published its International Classification of Sleep Disorders in 2005. The categories of childhood sleep disorder are given below, with some suggestions for how to overcome them. They are considered disorders only when they persist for a prolonged period of time and significantly disrupt the sleep of both your child and you.

Sleep Onset Association Disorder This refers to when a child has learned to fall asleep only when certain conditions are present and only with your intervention – for example, if your baby falls asleep only if you're rocking or feeding him. During the night when your son or daughter experiences a "normal" awakening at the end of a sleep cycle, he or she isn't able to self-soothe back to sleep.

Solution: Encourage self-soothing. Put your baby to bed when he or she is drowsy but not fully asleep. For both babies and older children, use the "camping-out" method (see box, p.80).

Limit-setting Sleep Disorder This disorder occurs more frequently in pre-school age or older children and is characterized by your child refusing to go to bed, even when you repeatedly call for bedtime. It's estimated that between 10 and 15 percent of toddlers and pre-school children resist bedtime in this way.

Solution: It's never too late to establish a bedtime routine and to adhere to a strict bedtime. Schedule some wind-down and settling time to help him or her prepare for going to sleep. If routine isn't the problem, you need to be firm. Every time he or she gets out of bed, take your child back lovingly but without talking. Eventually children learn that it's very boring to resist. Occasionally, restless leg syndrome (see pp.178–80), asthma or certain medications can cause this disorder, so if you're concerned, see your doctor.

Adjustment Sleep Disorder This disorder (which occurs in adults, too, as adjustment insomnia; see pp.143–6) is often the result of stress or illness. It may appear when families move house, for example, and the child finds it hard to adjust to new surroundings.

Solution: Go back to basics – follow a clear pre-sleep routine and ensure that your child is going to bed tired or drowsy, but awake. If necessary, use the "camping out" method to restore feelings of security and with them a "normal" sleeping pattern.

Environmental Sleep Disorder Too much light or noise, being too warm or too cold, having a TV in the room, and so on, can all disturb a child's sleep, leading to this chronic sleep problem.

Solution: Read pages 42–5 on how to promote the best sleeping environment – the information is as relevant to your child as it is to you. Improve as many of these environmental factors as you can.

Inadequate Sleep Hygiene Good sleep hygiene promotes sleep by reducing environmental stimulation and increasing relaxation – without these triggers your child may find it difficult to go to sleep, both at bedtime and when he or she wakes up naturally during the night. New and unexpected events; anxiety; excessive noise, cold or heat; vigorous exercise; hunger or large meals; pain and so on – all such factors contribute to poor sleep hygiene in children.

Solution: Establish a pre-sleep routine. Plan bedtime activities carefully – choose those that have a calming influence. Story-telling may be a tranquil activity, but unfamiliar stories or books that make noises may be too stimulating. Try to keep bathtime softly lit, with gentle play rather than vigorous splashing. Save a special toy for cuddling at bedtime, or offer a comfort blanket that stays in the cot or bed so that its associations are only with sleep. And, just like adults, children need a comfortable bed within a secure, quiet environment at a cool temperature – layers of cellular blankets are better than duvets for babies and very young children.

CAMPING OUT

The following steps set out a version of the "camping out" method for encouraging a young child to sleep through the night.

1. Set up your baby's room so that you have a comfortable chair next to the cot. Place your baby in the cot while drowsy but still awake. Sit in the chair and gently stroke or pat the baby until he or she falls asleep. Avoid talking and eye contact, but do utter soothing "shhhh" sounds. If the baby wriggles out of his or her sleeping position, put him or her back gently, without talking.
2. Once your baby is asleep, creep out of the room. If he or she wakes during the night, repeat the patting and stroking without at any point lifting the baby out of the cot.
3. Once your baby has become used to falling asleep within a few minutes with you patting, stroking and saying "shhhh", repeat the process, this time without any physical contact – sit next to the cot and say "shhhh". This way the baby gets used to your reassuring physical presence and the soothing sounds, but without any actual touching. If the baby wakes in the night, sit beside the cot and soothe with a "shhhh". Increase the intervals between the first cry and the moment at which you go to soothe.
4. Once the baby is used to falling asleep this way, move the chair farther from the cot. Repeat step 3 from this increased distance. On each consecutive night, move the chair closer toward the door, until you can soothe from outside the room. During night wakings, soothe from your new position and again increase the intervals between the first cry and your response.
5. Be patient. It may take three or four weeks to get to the point at which your baby or young child goes to sleep without any reassurance from you and is able to sleep through the night (most babies will still have the odd blip).

Sleep training – getting it right

Training a baby or young child to sleep through the night can be a stressful experience for parents. Apart from wanting the best for the baby, parents need their sleep, too. In the very first weeks, allow the baby to sleep as and when he or she needs – and you should nap at those times, too. Once you reach the 8- to 12-week mark, though, you can start to teach your baby the difference between night and day and he or she may begin to respond accordingly.

It goes against our most basic human instincts to leave a baby to cry, although the "crying it out" method is one approach to teaching a baby to self-soothe. It utilizes a psychological method that is clinically known as "extinction" – if the baby gets no attention as a result of a certain behaviour, eventually he or she gives up and stops repeating the behaviour (in this case crying). The approach may seem harsh (certainly, there are strong arguments against using it) and it takes enormous will power on the part of the parents to persevere to the point of success. Many parents find controlled crying a more palatable way to overcome nighttime waking; or "camping out", which can be a lengthy process, but altogether less stressful and yet equally effective. See the box, opposite.

TEENS TO TWENTIES

In the world of sleep medicine, adolescence lasts from around 12 years old until the ages from 22 to 25. I doubt if many 25-year-olds would consider themselves "adolescent", but in sleep terms it takes this long for sleeping patterns to mature.

By the time children reach school age, and until they begin to enter puberty at around 12 years old, they need around ten hours sleep in every 24 hours to optimize their physical and mental functioning. At puberty, this need falls slightly, to just over nine hours sleep a night.

The problem is that at the same time the pubescent body clock begins to operate on a go-slow. During adolescence the body's circadian rhythms enter "phase delay". Melatonin secretion occurs much later than is "sensible" for someone who needs to clock up nine hours of sleep, but who also needs to get up early to go to school (or to work) five or six mornings out of seven. If you're a parent to a teenager, it may come as a relief to know that your apparently rebellious son or daughter is not staying up late as an act of defiance. Even if he or she went to bed at 9pm, they would probably still be awake at 11. Nor are teenagers simply lazy: having to be coerced out of bed on days when they have to go to school and sleeping in late at the weekends are merely the body's way to try to make up the sleep deficit when it can.

One recent study revealed that 85 percent of 14- to 16-year-olds make up their sleep debt at the weekend. Although this seems a sensible approach to making sure adolescents get enough sleep over the course of a week, failing to keep to regular sleeping and waking times affects overall sleep hygiene and exacerbates the underlying problem with the teenage body clock. It's much more important to try to keep to a regular sleep–wake cycle, both during the week and at weekends. Scientists have seen some success with light–dark therapy helping to reset the teenage biological clock. Have a look at the box opposite to see if its advice could help you.

Nonetheless, lack of sleep is a problem for so-called "tweens". In a study by the National Sleep Foundation of the USA in 2006, 70 percent of adolescents who said they felt unhappy or even depressed also reported that they weren't getting enough sleep. Whether the lack of sleep leads to a lowered mood or vice versa is the subject of much debate, but it's commonly accepted that tackling the sleep deficit by attempting to get nine hours sleep a night is the best way for adolescents to begin to lift their mood. Interestingly, boys tend to become more sleep-deprived than girls.

The busy teen

Of course, delayed melatonin secretion is not the only reason that teenagers and young adults don't get enough sleep. The adolescent lifestyle often makes the problem worse. After-school or after-work activities (from football to parties) may be responsible for late nights, especially during the school years when there's homework time to consider, too. Similarly, in-room TV and games consoles make the

SLEEP THERAPY

RESETTING THE CLOCK

In order to covercome the problems associated with phase delay, so that you are, or your teenager is, better able to go to bed at a reasonable time and not feel tired in the morning, try the following light-therapy exercise, which brings bedtime and the morning alarm forward in 15-minute increments. The following assumes the need to get up at 7am, and therefore go to bed at 10pm – your own timings will vary with age and circumstance. You'll need an alarm – ideally, a dawn simulation alarm clock (see Resources, p.208).

1. For the first morning, try to choose a day on which it's OK to get up at 8am – so perhaps a weekend rather than a school or work day. On the previous night, set the dawn alarm for 8am. Assuming that it's dark outside and you aren't bothered by the noise or streetlight, leave your curtains open. (If that's not possible, or if dawn would be earlier than 6am, ask a willing accomplice to open your curtains at 6am.) Go to bed at 11.30pm. Although this is too late in the long term, it's counterproductive to associate bed with wakefulness, so it's better to go to bed when there's a high probability that you'll go to sleep.

2. In the morning, get up *as soon as* either the dawn wakes you or the alarm goes off. Once you've begun to wake naturally before the alarm, bring your bedtime and your alarm time forward by 15 minutes – with bedtime at 11.15pm and the alarm set for 7.45am. Repeat the process until you've brought bedtime forward to 10pm and the alarm to 7am. By this point, you should have entrained your body to feel sleepy at ten, and wake naturally by seven. It may take time, but with perseverance (and an understanding teacher or boss), you'll get there.

bedroom a place of activity rather than a place conducive to rest. If a member of your family is finding it hard to sleep, make sure that the TV and games consoles are out of bounds for at least two hours before bedtime. Try to keep activity schedules within sensible levels – after-school or after-work clubs once or twice a week, as well as a single night out with friends on a Friday or Saturday, should be the most any adolescent should attempt during a single week if he or she wants to be able to get enough sleep, too.

The issues for lack of sleep

You might ask whether or not it really matters if a teenager or young adult has a sleep deficit. The answer is yes, it really does. Apart from the increased risk of sadness or depression, and the need to establish good sleeping habits by the onset of adulthood, adolescents who don't get enough sleep are also more likely to lack concentration, be more irritable or moody, be increasingly clumsy and hurt themselves, and fall asleep during classes or at work. Alarmingly, under-25s cause more than half the road–traffic accidents that occur in the USA as a direct result of the driver's sleepiness.

The solutions

If you're a parent, encourage your son or daughter into a weektime activity schedule that isn't crammed full with evening commitments. Encourage good sleep hygiene, including making sure they that have a bedtime routine and that they go to bed and get up at roughly the same times every day – even at the weekends.

Research shows that youngsters sleep less if they have a TV, computer or other gadget in their bedroom. If possible, keep all this gear out of the bedroom, but if you can't, then divide the room up so that the bed is clearly reserved for sleep only. Loft beds are great for this: the space underneath the bed becomes a "room" in itself, suitable for activity; while climbing the ladder to bed provides a physical barrier that demarcates the difference between waking space and sleeping space.

Teens with cell phones will often not be parted with them. Insist on the use of an app that acts as an alarm clock, but also can be set

SLEEP SCIENCE

SYNAPTIC PRUNING AND SLEEP

In 2004 the US Department of Health funded an investigation into how childrens' brainwaves change between the ages of 9 and 14, including while they sleep. It found that age (rather than any hormone release or "sexual maturation") triggers the onset of something called synaptic pruning – a process in which the brain's numerous synapses (the bridges that pass information from one neuron to another) are reorganized and pared down to adult levels. The result is a brain with fewer connections, but with a faster, more efficient and more powerful processor. This natural occurrence is thought to begin at around age 11, and coincides with a decline in delta-wave (deep) sleep. By the time children reach 14 years old, their deep sleep hours have reduced by around 25 percent. Although the same overall decline in deep sleep occurs in both boys and girls, girls tend to begin the process of brain maturation (and so loss of deep sleep) earlier than boys.

to automatically cut the link with the telephone network and WiFi. Alternatively, turn off the phone and use an app that monitors whether or not it is turned back on again.

If you're at the upper end of the "adolescent" age range, the same applies – but, assuming you have no on-hand parent to keep you in check, you simply need to be firm with yourself.

SLEEP AND OLDER AGE

Trying to categorize the changing quality of sleep over the course of life is as difficult as categorizing sleep itself. How we interpret the quality of our sleep has so much to do with what we expect from it that we first have to consider what the "norms" are for our stage in life. For example, a twenty-year-old who wakes early in the morning might say that he or she has had a bad night's sleep or is not getting enough sleep. When that same twenty-year-old reaches the age of seventy, early waking might seem normal and acceptable – the problem instead might be falling asleep or frequent wakings during the night.

As it is, age seems to affect only a few sleep variables, and the generalization that older people sleep for fewer hours because they need less sleep is simply untrue. In the general population older people may sleep less because of the various health burdens associated with advancing years (including pain that keeps them awake, problems with mobility that make turning difficult, having to go to the loo more often during the night and so on), but in extremely healthy people over the age of, say, sixty there's actually little to distinguish an older person's sleep from that of someone who is younger.

There are a few generalizations we can make, though, about sleep over the course of our lifetimes:

• Deep sleep is deepest in children.
• The biological clock tends to speed up a little as we age, which means that the elderly tend to feel sleepier and fall asleep earlier than the rest of the population – but that also means that they wake up earlier.
• The biological clock may have a less regular or weaker rhythm in older age – but we need further research to confirm this.
• Older people are less tolerant of jet lag or shift work…
• … but they are more tolerant of lack of sleep and sleep disruption.
• Although healthy older people retain the same levels of dreaming sleep as younger people, they remember fewer of their dreams, particularly their napping dreams.

The table opposite shows how sleep changes between the ages of 37 and over 70 years old in both men and women, by looking at each sleep stage as a percentage of the overall time asleep. This is known as your sleep "architecture". The table shows that the biggest difference over time occurs in men's sleep, with deep sleep reducing by almost half during the course of those 35 or more years.

Percentage of Time Spent in Sleep Stages							
	DROWSY SLEEP		LIGHT SLEEP		DEEP SLEEP		REM SLEEP
AGE (years)	men / women		men / women		men / women		men / women
37–54	6	5	61.	59	11	14	20	21
55–60	6	5	65	56	8	17	19	20
61–70	7	5	65	57	7	17	18	19
>70	8	5	67	57	6	17	18	19

Apart from the gender-specific sleep changes that both men and women go through as they age (see pp.90–101), there are similar issues for both sexes in their advancing years. In general, from around 35 to 40 years old (mid-life) to somewhere in the eighties, men and women see a decrease of around 30 minutes total sleep time for each decade that passes. This means that by the time we reach ninety years old, assuming we were getting eight hours in our younger years, we're sleeping for only around six hours a night.

In older age, we experience increased awakenings and arousals; and maintaining any particular sleep stage becomes more difficult. Although the reasons why this should happen are not entirely clear, we do know that the biggest sleep thief is illness (both psychiatric and physical). Research indicates that conditions such as arthritis, diabetes, stroke and osteoporosis don't contribute significantly to symptoms of insomnia, but obesity, bodily pain, depression, heart disease, lung disease and bladder problems do.

• Obesity contributes to waking up a lot during the night and waking in the morning feeling unrefreshed.
• Bodily pain, depression and heart disease inhibit our ability to fall asleep, and cause us to wake frequently during the night, wake too early, and wake feeling unrefreshed.
• Lung disease may lead to feelings of tiredness in the morning.
• Memory problems are associated with difficulty in falling asleep and frequent wakings during the night.
• Nocturia (going to the loo several times during the night) and

increased blood pressure and bladder urgency cause frequent nighttime wakings.

On the other hand, difficulty sleeping may itself cause some of these age-related ailments, and others. For example:
• Snoring may lead to obesity and pain.
• Cessation in breathing (sleep apnoea) may cause obesity, lung disease and depression.
• Restless legs may lead to pain, depression and stroke.
• Daytime sleepiness may result in obesity, pain, depression, lung disease and memory problems.

The effects of poor-quality sleep

Getting fewer hours sleep can become a serious problem among the older generation. The reduction in sleep time leads to impaired mood and fewer hours spent in physical activity. In turn, older people may spend less time socializing with others (exacerbating psychiatric problems) and will find that their airways can weaken through lack of exercise, which only makes worse any sleep-related breathing disorders (see pp.170–74).

Getting help

Many older people don't report their sleep problems to their doctor, considering it a normal sign of ageing. I've also found that older people are more likely to self-medicate, using over-the-counter sleep aids, or an alcoholic nightcap. It probably goes without saying that I recommend neither of these. (In particular, bear in mind that if you take sleeping pills and suffer from nocturia, you're at an increased chance of falling when you get up in the night to go to the loo.)

Instead, it's important to work with your body, age and stage of life to optimize your sleeping hours. Keep to a regular schedule – get up at the same time each day, try to spend at least 30 minutes in physical activity (walking and doing the cleaning or gardening all count), and go out and get as much natural light as you can. Late afternoon and early evening are good times to be outdoors. The natural light then

SLEEP CLINIC

My elderly mother claims that she needs her "nana nap" every day, but then complains that she can't sleep at night. Is the nap the problem?

Elderly people do seem to nap more, but why this should be the case is not clear. Of the minimal amount of research that we've conducted, severe sleep-related breathing disorders (see pp.170–74) appear to have the biggest impact on feelings of daytime sleepiness and therefore the need to nap. Whether or not the naps are good or bad remains the subject of much debate. On the good side, it seems they may help cardiovascular health, and improve daytime function, and may even improve nighttime sleep. In fact, evidence suggests that poor nighttime sleep in the elderly is more likely down to breathing disorders than to any daytime napping.

Be aware, though, that while it's good for her to catch up on her sleep, napping may increase her chances of falling (owing to grogginess as she comes round) and of ischaemic heart disease, and it may indicate cognitive decline. Keep an eye on her – but certainly don't prevent her from napping if she feels she needs it.

helps to keep your circadian rhythms in tune with real time, potentially easing symptoms of phase advance (the need to go to sleep early). Of course, avoid caffeine, alcohol and other stimulant drinks before bedtime. If you need to nap in the afternoon, take your nap as soon as you can after lunch and restrict it to 20 to 30 minutes in duration.

Try not to fall asleep in front of the TV during the evening and use the relaxation exercises in this book to help to prepare your body for sleep each night. Also, bear in mind that medications you may be taking for other ailments may affect your sleep. Sometimes a change of dosage or a shift in the time you take your medication can improve your sleep at night. However, never make any changes without discussing them first with your medical practitioner.

Finally, don't simply assume that because you're getting older, you have to accept feeling unrefreshed every day. Talk to your doctor if lack of nighttime sleep is affecting how you feel and what you can do. Ensure that you receive the help and support you need to get some good-quality sleep at any and every age.

SLEEPING BEAUTY, SLEEPING LION

Anyone who has ever shared a bed with a member of the opposite sex will undoubtedly know that the sleep of men and women don't always coexist seamlessly. There are certain periods in a woman's or a man's life that particularly affect sleep. Menstruation, pregnancy and menopause can have a dramatic effect on a woman's sleeping patterns; while the sleep of men is particularly affected by ageing.

The differences between the sleeping patterns of men and of women begin at infancy and are intrinsic to every cell in the male and female body. Male and female genes have different impact on breathing control, the way the biological clock responds to stress, the function of the hypothalamus (the region of the brain that links the nervous system to the endocrine system, which governs the body's release of hormones) and even how cells grow and die.

Using an actigraph – a device that monitors gross motor movement and attaches to the wrist like a watch – to measure how much a subject moves around during sleep reveals that infant boys are likely to be poorer sleepers than infant girls. It also shows that, with age, girls seem to take longer to get to sleep, but once they've nodded off are more likely to sleep longer than boys. By adolescence, girls' sleep is longer and more efficient than boys'. An EEG shows that, at birth, the oscillations of boys' slow-wave (deep) sleep are particularly slow, but that by adulthood (which for sleep is in the twenties; see p.81) women have "better" slow-wave sleep than men.

Women and sleep

In general, women need around 20 minutes more sleep than men in every 24-hour period. No one is certain why this would be, but some scientists at Loughborough University in the UK have hypothesized that in order to perform multiple, complex tasks simultaneously, women use more of their brains than men do, so they have increased need for consolidation time – and that means a greater need for sleep.

Objectively, girls and women sleep better and longer than men – subjectively, however, women are more likely to complain of insomnia. A study by the University of North Carolina has shown that women are more likely to rack up a sleep debt than men are. This finding is compounded by a study in Canada in which 35 percent of women said they have trouble sleeping, compared with only 25 percent of men. Women tend to be lighter sleepers, disturbed more easily during the night than men. For example, a woman is more likely to rouse at the mere whisper of her name or the gentle snuffles of her baby. A fidgety partner is more likely to bring her round from sleep completely. To make matters worse, a study at the University of Surrey, UK, has shown that once roused, women find it harder to get back to sleep.

Sleep and the menstrual cycle

Why is it that women are more likely to sleep badly? As with so much about sleep, we don't yet have concrete answers. However, it's likely that women worry more than men. They are also more emotional, finding it harder to switch off. But there could be physiological reasons, too. During the menstrual cycle, at the point at which the egg has been released from the ovarian follicle and the remnants of the follicle have released the hormone progesterone, a woman's temperature might rise by up to 0.4°C (32.7°F). This slight increase can make a woman feel too hot in bed, making it harder to get to sleep or to stay asleep.

The menstrual cycle also disrupts a woman's rhythms for releasing melatonin, thyroid-stimulating hormone and cortisol. Frustratingly, research is not clear as to the impact of these disruptions on major sleep characteristics (the amount of deep sleep, dreaming sleep and so on a woman has), but we do know that there are subtle effects at work. For example, at certain stages of the menstrual cycle, a woman has a greater abundance of sleep spindles in the upper frequencies, although we don't actually know yet what this means for women in practical terms. On the whole, though, while women without other menstrual difficulties may complain of lighter sleep around the time of menstruation, the impact on sleep of the differing hormonal milieu appears to be minimal. If you suffer from PMS or PCOS, however, you may have a different story to tell (see box, pages 94–5).

Of course, it's not just the menstrual cycle that uniquely affects female sleep. Pregnancy and menopause are times when sleep patterns go through changes that are exceptional to any other time in a woman's life.

Sleep and pregnancy

I've often heard mothers say that lack of sleep during pregnancy is the body's way to prepare a woman for the first few sleep-deprived months of new parenthood. I don't know if that's true, but from a weak bladder to sleeping with a bump, there are many aspects of pregnancy that conspire to make restorative sleep much longed for.

Studies indicate that women who are having their first babies suffer greater sleep deprivation than those in their second or subsequent pregnancies. This suggests that apart from the physical reasons why a pregnant woman might have less good-quality sleep (which affects all women in pregnancy, regardless of how many babies they've had), there are psychological factors at work, too – such as anxiety about the baby or birth. In general, research suggests that pregnant women have less deep sleep, and less dreaming and more drowsy sleep than non-pregnant women. There's some evidence to suggest that lack of sleep during pregnancy may lead to pre-term delivery or may increase your chances of suffering post-natal depression. For these reasons, and for your own ability to cope with the demands of pregnancy, it's important to do everything you can to optimize your chances of sleeping well while you're carrying a baby.

Pregnancy is divided into three "trimesters". The first occurs from conception to three months, the second from four to six months, and the third from seven months until birth. In a study of 300 pregnant women, the rate of nighttime awakenings increased by 63 percent in the first trimester, 80 percent in the second and 84 percent in the third, suggesting that insomnia develops with the developing baby.

Sleep during the first trimester

From the moment of her baby's conception, a woman's body goes through innumerable hormonal changes aimed at ensuring she carries her baby to term. Some of these hormones increase the blood-flow through the body by up to a third, while increases in progesterone (up to 5,000 times pre-pregnancy levels) relax the smooth muscles of the bladder. This means that on the one hand more blood is being flushed through the kidneys, creating more waste (urine), and on the other, the bladder itself is "weaker". Finally, a growing uterus within the pelvis in the first three months of pregnancy begins to put pressure on the bladder, which in turn increases how often the bladder feels full. The result is that both during the day and during the night, a woman in early pregnancy needs far more trips to the loo. At night, this can significantly disrupt a good night's sleep.

The best way to try to minimize nighttime trips to the loo is to ensure that you get the majority of your fluids before 7pm in the evening. Avoid tea, coffee and alcohol in the evening altogether – you should in any case drink these to a minimum while you're pregnant. All these drinks are diuretic, which means that they pass through your system quickly and increase the need to urinate.

Sleep during the second trimester

Between four and six months of pregnancy, hormone levels settle down and the uterus moves out of the pelvis to make space for the growing baby, temporarily relieving pressure on the bladder. This is probably the time in your pregnancy when you're least likely to need the loo in the night. However, other things conspire to disrupt sleep.

You may experience leg cramps, a blocked nose, and strange and vivid dreams (see box, p.97). Note that a blocked nose (which may cause you to snore) can be a sign of increased blood pressure, so make sure you mention it to your doctor or midwife. Some studies claim that your sleeping position can affect the health of your baby. Avoid sleeping on your back after 16 weeks of pregnancy, as the weight of the baby can put pressure on your blood vessels, and sleep on your left side to increase the blood-flow through the baby. However, if you

PMS, PCOS AND SLEEP

Almost a quarter of all women suffer from premenstrual syndrome (PMS) – including period pain and mood disorders – and/or polycystic ovary syndrome (PCOS). These women are generally two to three times more likely to experience excessive sleepiness in the daytime and insomnia at night during their menstrual cycle.

If you have PMS

At night, you may find that you move around more, and are likely to wake up more frequently and suffer disturbing dreams. During the daytime, you may have increased fatigue and sleepiness and reduced concentration. Your parasympathetic nervous system, which regulates your bodily functions during sleep (see pp.31–5), may stop working properly, reducing the restorative power of sleep. During sleep your pain threshold lowers, so if you suffer from dysmenorrhoea (period pain) at night, your cramps will feel particularly uncomfortable, waking you or keeping you awake.

Your best strategy is to manage the effects of PMS – and there are many wonderful books dedicated to this subject, which is too involved to do justice to here. In the case of period pain, though, I do recommend taking a painkiller such as ibuprofen or paracetamol (if they are not contraindicated) before you go to bed, as well as a non-steroidal anti-inflammatory, at least until you've managed your symptoms in other ways.

If you have PCOS

Polycystic ovary syndrome is caused by hormonal imbalance. It occurs when follicles on the surface of the ovaries fail to develop and wither away properly, causing cysts. It can contribute to chronic period pain and exacerbate all the symptoms of PMS.

Independently, though, it's been linked with increased sleep-related breathing disorders, such as sleep apnoea (see pp.170–78). Many women with PCOS are given the contraceptive pill to help regulate the hormone levels throughout their cycle and so reduce the condition's effects, including its effects on sleep. However, bear in mind that this in itself can affect your sleep (see box, below). Women with PCOS are also prone to weight gain. If you develop a breathing disorder, bear in mind that losing weight (if appropriate) may help to ease the symptoms.

SLEEP CLINIC

Since I've begun taking the contraceptive pill I feel far less refreshed after sleeping. Is there a link?

Studies show that oral contraceptives reduce the amount of deep sleep women get and increase the amount of light sleep. They also increase body temperature throughout the menstrual cycle (and even for a while after you stop taking the Pill). Some research suggests that the oral contraceptive influences or inhibits the body's melatonin secretion – but so far the results are inconclusive. In short, it is indeed likely that now you're taking the Pill you're experiencing some sleep problems. As an initial step, try keeping your bedroom a little cooler to see if you can counter the effects of your raised temperature. If you feel that your sleep is becoming significantly compromised, see your doctor and perhaps even consider alternative methods of contraception.

wake up and find yourself on your back or on your right side, don't fret – simply turn over. If you're worried that you'll turn in your sleep, putting a pillow behind your back as you lie on your left can help you stay in position. Keep your knees pulled up toward your bump. If your hips begin to ache (which may be caused by the loosening of the ligaments around your pelvis), sleep with a pillow between your knees.

Stick to your sleep hygiene routine, including going to bed and getting up at the usual times. Give yourself the luxury of an afternoon nap if you need to – but keep it short (not more than 20 to 30 minutes) and make it early in the afternoon.

Sleep during the third trimester

More than half of all pregnant women claim that their sleep is worst of all during the third trimester of pregnancy.

As the baby grows bigger, your uterus expands further so that it again fills the space in your pelvis and puts pressure on your bladder. Unfortunately, therefore, the frequent nighttime trips to the loo may make a reappearance. Lean forward as you pee, which will help you to empty your bladder fully.

Your bump is also going to make it increasingly difficult for you to find a comfortable sleeping position. Stick to sleeping on your left side, with a pillow between your knees if it helps and one under your bump to help support it. If lying down is just completely uncomfortable, you may find it easier to sleep propped up in bed instead.

It's common to experience heartburn at this time, too, as there's little space in your stomach for food, while the high levels of progesterone relax the muscles of the oesophagus, making it easier for food to come back up. Avoid rich or spicy foods at the end of the day, which may anyway cause heartburn, and try to eat little and often rather than opting for one main meal in the evening. Again, sleeping propped up can help alleviate the heartburn.

More than a quarter of pregnant women in their third trimester may suffer Restless Leg Syndrome – the feeling that creepy crawlies are climbing your legs so that you feel a constant need to move your legs to relieve the sensation. This is particularly marked in women in

SLEEP CLINIC

I'm just past my first trimester and since I got pregnant I've been having extremely vivid dreams. Is this normal?

Yes, it's completely normal! Your body is going through an intense period of change. You're also acutely aware that your life is about turn on its head – or at least that's what people tell you. Your dreams are an outlet for your anxieties. The journey to parenthood is one of the most exhilarating but also daunting you're ever likely to face, so it's to be expected that you try to unravel your feelings about it during your sleep. You'll probably keep having vivid dreams right up until the point you have the baby – although their content might change. In the early days of pregnancy, many women dream about giving birth to baby animals, or have dreams that represent anxieties about their changing shape. In a Swiss study, 17 percent of women in their second trimester reported an increase in erotic dreams. Some experts think that this is the woman's way to reassure herself that she's still attractive. Toward the end of the third trimester, dreams may focus on anxieties about childbirth or meeting the baby for the first time.

Keep a dream diary. Not only will this offer you an outlet for expressing your dreams and your emotions during your waking hours, it's also a wonderful record to show to your baby when he or she is older. (You might want to leave out the erotica, though!)

their first pregnancy. Read my advice for overcoming this disorder on pages 178–80, but bear in mind that the condition is associated with low iron. Increasing your intake of folate-rich foods can help – lentils, beans, pulses and spinach are all good sources. Vitamin-C-rich foods will enable your body to absorb the folate more efficiently. Check with your doctor or midwife, but iron and folate supplements can help, too.

Finally, many women say that their baby seems to "wake up", dancing around in the uterus, the moment they try to sleep. There's debate as to whether or not it's true that babies in the womb work on a nocturnal cycle, or whether it's simply that when the mother is still, the baby's movements are more noticeable. Even so, there's very little you can do about this except to try to change your thinking patterns so that rather than becoming a source of irritation and sleeplessness, your baby's movements feel reassuring to you that all is well.

Above all, remember that lack of sleep might feel dreadful for you but it doesn't harm your baby in any way. Do your best to rest as much as you can during the day (although remember the note about napping, on page 96). You may find that relaxation techniques or classes (such as antenatal pilates or yoga) help to give you a pervading sense of calm, making sleep more likely. You can also try a bedtime relaxation, to put you in the mood for sleep, such as the Humming Bee Breath meditation on page 71.

Menopause and sleep

In the West, menopause typically occurs any time between the ages of 40 and 58 years old (on average at around 51 years old). The timing depends upon a variety of factors, including your ethnicity, how old you were when you had children, whether you breastfed, and your weight. The signs of approaching menopause – at first irregular periods, then later, intermittent periods, hot flushes, loss of libido, and mood swings among them – may be evident several years before a woman ceases to menstruate altogether. This lead time is called the "peri-menopause".

There are very few objective studies on the effects of menopause, but those that have been conducted offer some insight into how the menopause, and its side effects, may inhibit good-quality sleep. One study noted that during the first half of the night, women with hot flushes had significantly more arousals and awakenings than a control group and those without hot flushes. Women who were convinced that their hot flushes were causing a problem with their sleep on average reported around five hot flushes per night, and five sleep disturbances. Interestingly, the awakenings occurred immediately before each hot flush. In trying to find a solution to the problem, the researchers found that a lower ambient temperature of 18°C (64.5°F), compared with

20°C and 23°C (68°F and 73.4°F), reduced the number of hot flushes in susceptible women by 25 percent. I think 18°C is about the right room temperature (if such a generalization can be made) for sleep anyway (see p.46), so you may need to go cooler than this to see an improvement in your symptoms.

Furthermore, oestrogen is believed to have an impact on the biological clock, making it harder to fall asleep or causing you to wake too early in the morning. However, we need much more research in this area to be able to make conclusive statements about the link between the two. Oestrogen is also thought to affect the size of your thermo-neutral zone – the temperature zone in which sleep is comfortable and undisturbed. As women stop producing oestrogen with the onset of the menopause, so their tolerance of temperature diminishes. This means that your optimal sleeping temperature before you began entering the menopause may now seem stiflingly hot, exacerbating your susceptibility to hot flushes and night sweats. As there's little you can do to increase your oestrogen levels again, try to eliminate or overcome any of the other things that reduce your tolerance to temperature. These include smoking, physical inactivity and being overweight.

Men and sleep

Men present something of an anomaly to sleep science. On the one hand, they're less likely to report tiredness and disturbed sleep than women are; but on the other they show far more sleep abnormalities when their sleep is recorded at a sleep centre. Why would this be? Perhaps it's simply that women are far more willing to share their problems (we know that in other areas of medicine women are more likely to tell you when they are, for example, depressed or anxious). Or is it something else?

Men more often suffer from obstructive sleep apnoea than women – which is probably why men are more often accused of snoring. Sleep apnoea is likely to cause increased daytime sleepiness, but also shortens the time it takes a sufferer to fall asleep. Even though the sleep disorder is pathological (the result of a physical defect), sufferers are likely to report that they "sleep like a log", feeling that falling asleep comes easily to them and without making the association that daytime sleepiness might in fact be because their nighttime sleep is interrupted by momentary lapses in breathing.

In men it's particularly noticeable that poor sleep causes problems with glucose control, which in turn is associated with the development of increased blood pressure – and therefore heart attack and stroke. The precise reasons why this happens are not clear, but the signs are that sleep disruption and restriction have direct effects on the body's inflammatory mechanism – which conspires to cause thickening of the arteries and vascular disease. The physical effects are then compounded by the fact that feeling sleepy during the day inevitably means doing less exercise; while low glucose levels mean that men are more likely to seek out a sugar hit to give them a boost of energy. A diet high in refined sugar is linked with obesity, itself a cause of heart disease – and sleep apnoea. And so the cycle goes on.

Although it's important that men who are overweight and suffer from sleep apnoea take steps to lose weight (see p.174), unfortunately this will not necessarily spell the end for their sleep-related breathing disorder. We think that this is because either long-term inflammation or damage to the neuromuscular control mechanisms of the neck prevents a return to normal breathing.

The most important thing you can do if you think you're overly sleepy during the day – even if you think you sleep well at night – is to go through all the steps relating to good sleep hygiene (see Chapter 3) to ensure the quality of your sleep is as good as it can be. Go to bed relatively early, perhaps 30 minutes to an hour before you think you need to. If you wake feeling refreshed, and you don't feel abnormally tired over the course of the day, you're doing OK.

Testosterone and sleep

Finally, a word about testosterone levels when men get too few hours sleep. Testosterone is commonly thought of as the "male" hormone, playing a key role in the development of the gender-specific traits of a man – the growth of the testes and prostate, as well as physical strength and bone density. Women also have some testosterone, but at much lower levels. A study at the University of Chicago in 2011 revealed that lack of sleep dramatically reduces male levels of testosterone – which can further increase a man's susceptibility to sleep-related breathing disorders and to obesity, not to mention its effects on erectile dysfunction and hypogonadism (when the gonads stop producing hormones properly).

CHAPTER 5

GOOD SLEEP GUIDES FOR WORKERS, PARENTS, DREAMERS AND MORE

Genetic make-up, our environment, and our health, age and gender, as well as our overall approach to sleep hygiene all affect our sleep. We can talk about the "average" person and their "average" sleep, but each of us is unique, facing our own sleep challenges. In this chapter, I take some of life's occupations and preoccupations and look specifically at how, if one of them applies to you, you can either overcome the issues your situation poses for your sleep, or use your sleep to help you to improve performance and ability in your waking life.

Dancer or dreamer, frequent flyer or long-distance driver, this chapter offers specific advice for specific circumstances.

A WORKER'S GUIDE TO GOOD SLEEP
What effects do lack of sleep have on your ability to work effectively? As we already know, disturbed sleep inhibits your attention span, your complex thinking skills and your ability to make good decisions. It may damage your social interactions and exacerbate inappropriate behaviours, because lack of good-quality sleep makes you more

impulsive. Furthermore, your colleagues will be able to tell from your appearance when you haven't had enough sleep. One study randomly selected half the members of a study group to have a bad night's sleep, asking the remainder to sleep well. The test was repeated with a new random selection on another night. On both occasions a panel of judges noticed simply by appearance which participants had had the good night and which had had the bad. You can't hide lack of sleep!

So, if your work involves looking good, feeling sharp-witted, and liaising collaboratively with others, getting a good night's sleep and reducing daytime sleepiness are essential.

What you can do
1. Optimize your sleep time

First and foremost make sure you give yourself the opportunity to get enough sleep. Calculate backwards from the time you need to leave your home to establish what time you need to go to bed. So:

- What time do you need to leave for work? (Say, 8am.)
- Deduct the time it takes for you to have your breakfast
  (say 30 minutes, giving 7.30am).
- Deduct the time it takes you to wash and dress
  (say 40 minutes, giving 6.50am).
- Deduct the amount of sleep you need in order to wake feeling
  refreshed (say, 7½ hours, giving 11.20pm).
- Deduct a further ten minutes so that you wake ten minutes
  before you absolutely have to get up (giving 11.10pm).
- Deduct the amount of time it usually takes you to fall asleep
  (say, 15 minutes, giving 10.55pm).

The time you need to be in bed with the light out is 10.55pm. Begin your bedtime routine (see pp.59–64) with this time in mind.

2. Release residual stress

All jobs come with their quota of stress. Many of the people I meet carry home that stress and mull it over in the hours of darkness. To give yourself the best possible chance for a good night's sleep, it's really important that you release residual anxiety before you go to bed. Read pages 69–72, which are specifically related to this subject, but also make sure that you have dealt with the day's "anxiety hangover" before you go to bed. The following make good strategies for work-related stress relief; use any or all of them as relevant.

- If you use public transport to get home, amend your journey so that you can build in a 15-minute walk before you step over the threshold. This might mean walking rather than driving home from the station, or getting off the bus one stop early. The pause between work and home helps to clear your head and the walk will give you a good burst of fresh air (and, in the summer, daylight) to help you fall asleep more easily later.

- Write a list of things you need to achieve tomorrow at work (beginning with any that didn't get done today) and put it in your work bag or case. Close the bag; no need to think about any of them now – you can deal with them tomorrow.

- If you had a difficult meeting or conversation over the course of the day and it's troubling you, make sure you talk it through with a partner or friend; or write a letter to yourself outlining brief details and what it is about the conversation or meeting that has upset you. Try to come up with three action points to recover or move forward the situation – which you can do tomorrow. Now, let the episode go for the day, knowing you have a plan for resolution in place. You can also use this technique if you're worried about something you know you have to do the following day.

3. Keep your energy levels stable

An adequate breakfast not only enables you to perform more efficiently during the day, it also reduces your chances of putting on weight, and a healthy weight improves your sleep. Breakfast is exactly what it says – a break in a natural fast. For this reason your brain likes carbohydrates in the morning to give it a good energy boost. Adding low-glycaemic index foods helps to release the carbohydrates slowly so that you don't feel hungry until lunchtime, and you don't feel as though you need a sugar fix to give you a bit of mid-morning zing. If you balance your breakfast with protein, too, studies show that you will find multi-tasking much easier. I encourage a morning cup of caffeinated coffee – I think it improves alertness and mental performance.

Make lunch protein-rich, with only small amounts of carbohydrate (see p.65), helping to keep your blood sugars stable over the course of the afternoon to attenuate mid-afternoon sleepiness. Avoid alcohol at lunchtime, too. Note that the mid-afternoon energy dip will get more pronounced as you grow older. If you aren't overly sensitive to caffeine, a 2.30pm cup of caffeinated coffee or tea will help stave off mental fatigue and shouldn't affect your nighttime sleep. However, avoid this if you do think it will keep you awake later.

Overall, make sure your diet contains sufficient amounts of iron (from green leafy vegetables, whole grains and cereals, as well as from red meat), as good levels of iron help to prevent daytime fatigue. Remember that vitamin-C-rich foods, such as oranges and grapefruits, help with iron absorption.

Try to ensure your day is broken up with a variety of tasks. That way, if you do get a sleepy period while you're at work, you can switch to something new to do, which can have an instantly invigorating effect on your energy levels.

A SHIFT WORKER'S GUIDE TO GOOD SLEEP

Shift work, especially when it involves nightshifts, has become the subject of much debate within the sleep community. We define shift work as any job that falls outside a 9.30am to 5.30pm (or thereabouts) working-hours routine. For many years sleep researchers have tried to unravel the effects of working shifts on health and well-being. However, empirical studies are skewed by the fact that those doing shift work are already more physiologically and psychologically able to cope with its demands, simply by virtue of their genetic make-up. We find that those unsuited to shift work leave their professions quickly once the erratic hours begin to take their toll. Those left for us to study don't, therefore, represent a true cross-section of the population.

Nevertheless, the major detrimental effects of shift work have over time become apparent. For women, studies reveal that shift work can increase susceptibility to breast cancer, and both sexes are more prone to gastrointestinal problems, increased blood pressure, and stroke. Night workers (including nurses, doctors and factory workers) are five times more likely to have a road-traffic accident on their way home at the end of their shift. What we're not clear about yet is what exactly causes the problems. Could it be fewer hours asleep (which we know is true of shift workers)? Disruption to the 24-hour biological clock? Or simply changes to lifestyle (for example, we know that nurses don't follow the same principles of a healthy lifestyle – nutritious diet, moderate, regular exercise and so on – that they ask of their patients). Furthermore, shift workers more often complain of insomnia, fatigue, lack of concentration, irritability and clumsiness. If you have any combination of these symptoms and you work shifts, you may have what is now termed "shift work sleep disorder".

What you can do

Although some literature suggests that there's a "perfect" rota scheme, in fact chronobiologists and sleep scientists agree that no shift-working rota can meet an ideal. Even in general terms it's hard to establish a best practice. However, if there's a consensus it's that shifts that follow a day-evening-night rotation are better than day-night-evening – probably because the former follows the direction of the body clock.

If you're a shift-worker and want to get the best out of your sleep, so that you can get the best out of your waking hours, both at work and at home, try to follow a few basic principles:

• Sleep whenever you can, even if this is in short two-hour bursts. Your body will ensure that you maximize the time you spend in deep, restorative sleep, and also in dreaming sleep. Also, don't be afraid to take naps during your shift breaks if you need to. Talk to your manager to try to ensure there's somewhere you can go to sit and shut your eyes for 20 minutes (but 20 minutes is enough). Now that we live in a 24/7 culture, workplaces are becoming much more aware and tolerant of the need to look after their night shifters.

- Try to keep your biological clock on a "normal" 24-hour schedule. One of the simplest ways to do this is to eat according to the usual schedule of a morning breakfast (keep it fairly small and carbohydrate-rich), a light lunch in the middle of the day and a main meal at supper time. If you're working a night shift, you'll need light snacks to keep you going – but be careful how you choose them (see box, p.108).
- Maintain your exercise levels. Making sure you do 30 minutes of exercise every day helps to keep you healthy and reduce the risks associated with shift work and/or obesity. Try to perform your 30 minutes (or more) at roughly the same time every day – even on your days off.
- Avoid caffeine and any other stimulation (including vigorous exercise) just before you intend to sleep.
- Read Chapter 3 on sleep hygiene and follow its advice as carefully as you can. Take special care to keep your bedroom dark, at the right temperature and for sleeping (and sex) only. Winding down and setting a bedtime routine is also especially important – your brain needs lots of triggers that it's time to sleep (see below).

Timing your sleep

Try to identify a particular period in every 24 hours when you're always asleep. Routine helps your body adjust to the constant changes to your working/sleeping patterns. Unfortunately, in order to maintain the new rhythm, you should also commit to sleeping at that time during your days off. So, for example, if your shift usually begins at 11pm and finishes at 7am, you should ideally make sure that you're asleep between the hours of 8am and 11am, every day.

If your shifts work on a rota system, keep to your given "sleep hours" as closely as you can throughout the rota. You might need to work out carefully which hours will always be your sleep hours, but usually the system can work, give or take 30 to 60 minutes.

SLEEP CLINIC

I work night shifts and find that the only way I can get through them is to snack on chocolate bars. It's not helping my waistline! What can I do?

First and foremost, make sure that you're eating healthily during the day. This means avoiding high-fat, spicy, and salty foods, and also doing your best to eat as though you were not working on shifts (see main text) – remember that in the middle of the night your digestive system slows down. If you've eaten well during the day, you shouldn't need to fill up on energy during your shift, although inevitably being active will occasionally make you feel peckish. Take healthy snacks with you into work – fruit, nuts and seeds, or a light salad will fill a hunger gap so that you're less tempted to reach for the sugar.

Drink lots of water, too, so that you feel less like you need sugar to keep going. Finally, if you feel sleepy early on in your shift, have a caffeinated drink. Although it's not good to drink caffeine shortly before trying to sleep, caffeine at the start of a nightshift shouldn't affect your ability to sleep later.

A final tip

It may help to wear sunglasses on your way home from work (as long as it doesn't make travelling dangerous). Reducing the amount of sunlight in your eyes in the morning helps slow down the cessation in melatonin secretion that tells your body it's time to wake up (just at the time that you need to be thinking about sleep).

A DRIVER'S GUIDE TO GOOD SLEEP

From truck drivers to sales people, there are many workers who drive long distances on a regular basis, sometimes sleeping in unfamiliar places in between. With more than a quarter of Americans admitting that they regularly drive when they feel sleepy, there's never been a greater need for some tips on how to ensure you can drive with full alertness, and what to do when you feel sleepy at the wheel.

In the UK in the 1960s, the British Highways Agency opened a number of motorways that traversed the country, with the aim that drivers could avoid snarled-up towns and instead use fast routes, particularly out of London. Before long the Automobile Association – a private support network for motorists – noticed that there were more accidents in the Lake District (in the north of England) in which characteristically the driver did not appear to take any action that would avoid the accident, nor reduce his or her speed before colliding with a stationary object. It turned out that in many cases the drivers had started their journey in London – leading to the conclusion that they had fallen asleep at the wheel. With such stark evidence for the dangers of driving when tired, the Government immediately introduced measures to try to ensure that motorists took alertness seriously.

As far as the law is concerned, a driver has a responsibility to drive safely – there can be no excuse for falling asleep nor even a lapse in attention. Nonetheless, in the USA it's thought that over a quarter of a million drivers may fall asleep at the wheel every day, and falling asleep while driving may lead to around 40,000 US deaths every year.

Danger zones

There are two predictable circumstances in which you are at greater risk of falling asleep at the wheel. Think of these as the driving "danger zones" and avoid them at all costs.

1. Time

Sleep-related motoring accidents are most likely to occur at two particular times of the night and day – even if you've had adequate sleep the night before your drive or you're driving only a short distance. The first is at 4am, when your biological clock has turned your body to its furthest point from waking alertness. The second most likely time is during the afternoon, at your natural post-lunch energy dip (older drivers particularly are most likely to have an accident at this time).

2. *Boredom*

Monotony increases sleepiness and that's why sleep-related crashes occur more frequently when we're driving on fast, long single- or dual-carriage roads, or on motorways or highways.

Sleep deficit effects

There's nothing complicated about the links between the amount of sleep you get and the risks associated with driving a car – the greater your sleep deficit, the higher your chances of being involved in a driving incident. It's important to remember that you needn't necessarily fall completely asleep to cause an accident. Falling asleep means closing your eyes, but before that point you may become drowsy and experience microsleeps. These are a mixture of sleep and wakefulness, lasting between three and ten seconds each – the longer they are, the more likely you are to perceive or remember them. Under normal circumstances – for example, when you're in bed – microsleeps lead to sleep, and laboratory experiments show without doubt that, if they happen when you're doing something active, they cause errors in judgment and response. In driving simulation this usually means reduced ability to control steering. The message is simple and clear (and in many countries is now part of the law): if you're driving and you feel you're *becoming* sleepy, you must pull over.

What you can do

Listening to music, driving with the windows open and so on might help you feel more alert for a bit, but they won't prevent you from falling asleep. The following are actions to take both during an emergency situation (such as when you hear the "rumble strips" because you've veered into the hard shoulder) and when you know that you have a long, boring journey ahead of you so need to prepare to stay awake.

In an emergency:

If you're driving, hear the sound of your tyres on the rumble strips and realize that you can't remember actively driving moments beforehand, you need to take an emergency break.

- Stop driving – pull over as soon as it is safe and legal to do so, ideally in a service station.
- Have a cup of caffeinated coffee and then take a nap or rest with your eyes closed for 15 to 20 minutes (your body will absorb the coffee while you nap). You should need to do this only once during your journey. If you need to nap more than once, you must try to find a hotel so that you can stop altogether for the day (or night). Remember to allow 10 to 15 minutes after your nap to become fully alert before driving again, and note that you shouldn't use caffeine to keep awake on long journeys or if you still have a long way to go, as the perceptible effects are short-lived.

For long journeys:

- Plan your journey and organize yourself before you set out. For example, avoid driving when you would normally be asleep and avoid driving during the nighttime and mid-afternoon danger zones (see p.109). Consider whether you could share the driving with someone else, taking the journey in two-hour shifts (giving you two-hour naps in the passenger seat). Ensure that the night before your drive, you optimize your chances of a good night's sleep and avoid alcohol or other drugs.
- Before you leave, work out where you might be able to stop overnight if you have to – and do stop. Your safety and the safety of other road users is *always* the priority.
- If you have a long stretch of any single road to drive along, consider whether or not you can re-route your journey so that you drive through a town or have to make several turns. This is a trade off – in the end it may you an extra half an hour, but you'll have forced yourself to be more alert. However, the longer journey may also increase your fatigue, in which case do what you know will work best for you.
- Plan for rest breaks every two hours and factor these in to your journey time. If you feel sleepy when you stop, take a nap for 20 minutes. Otherwise, get out of the car, stretch your legs and

get some fresh air. Obviously, if you feel sleepy before you hit two hours, stop as soon as possible.

• Keep a supply of caffeinated drinks and sugar-free chewing gum in the car with you (studies show that chewing gum can improve alertness in the short term).

A FLYER'S GUIDE TO GOOD SLEEP

In 2011, Chicago-based car salesman Thomas Stuker celebrated ten million air miles with United Airlines – he's thought to have flown more miles than any other passenger in history (although no one can be sure). He has spent his adult life frequently crossing time zones both within the USA and around the world. Of course, his story is exceptional, but generally more and more of us, on business and for pleasure, are travelling greater distances every year. But what are the effects on sleep both before and after time-zone travel, and how can we minimize them?

Studies show that there are three main factors that affect how a flyer feels when he or she arrives at a destination: jet lag, fatigue and stress.

Jet lag

Jet lag occurs when you move quickly from one time zone to another. Put simply, your travelling speed is faster than the speed of your internal 24-hour clock, so the clock doesn't have time to adjust before you reach your destination. It won't surprise you to know that there was never such a thing as "boat lag", when people travelled long distances slowly by sea. The symptoms of jet lag are fatigue, insomnia, restlessness, irritability, reduced appetite or feelings of nausea and altered bowel movements.

The world is divided up into 24 time zones, each equivalent to one hour of time. The zones are measured from a single point – Greenwich in London. From Greenwich, we add hours travelling eastward and take them away travelling westward. Generally, travelling somewhere that's between one and three hours ahead or behind your "home" time shouldn't cause any major difficulties, although this will partly depend

SLEEP CLINIC

I'm trying to plan how long I should make my business trip. How long will it take me to adjust?

As a rough rule of thumb, adapting to a new time zone can take as much as one day for each hour travelled westward (although often less than this), and one and a half days for each hour travelled eastward. Using light exposure and avoidance shortens this adjustment period considerably. It might surprise you to know that I recommend operating on your home time for the duration of your trip if you aren't travelling across more than six time zones and your trip is short – say only two or three days long. Although this can be awkward to manage if you have meetings, it does mean that you won't need your body to readapt twice (at your destination and when you get home) in a short period of time.

upon how sensitive you are to the demands of your biological clock. "Larks" (those people who bounce out of bed early in the morning; see box, p.17) tend to be a little more sensitive. If this is you, you may find that you have to take steps to reduce the effects of as little as three hours time difference.

All of us, however, tend to feel the effects of changing time zones if we add or take away four hours or more. Generally, we tend to find it easier to travel westward – to a time zone behind rather than ahead of our own. To set the biological clock back in time, the internal mechanism simply has to slow down more than it's used to. As a biological process this is easier than trying to speed it up. Given that most flights westward arrive during the day, it becomes fairly easy to get extra hours of daylight on arrival and in doing so slow down the biological clock so that it steps relatively quickly into rhythm with the new zone.

Furthermore, even if you arrive feeling sleepy, simply forcing yourself to stay up and awake helps the body's adjustment – you'll fall asleep

SLEEP SCIENCE

THE ARGONNE DIET

The US military uses a special diet, known as the Argonne Diet, to help soldiers readjust quickly to new time zones. Four days before a posting, the soldiers alternate feast and fast days, beginning with a feast day and ending with a fast day. During feast days they have no calorie limit and eat breakfasts and lunches that are high in protein and low in carbohydrate. Suppers are high in carbs and low in protein. Fasting days have an 800-calorie limit and consist of fruit for breakfast and lunch and vegetable soup for supper. The results are encouraging, as soldiers do seem better able to adjust quickly to their new time zone – up to seven times more quickly travelling westward and up to 16 times more quickly for eastward journeys. In my own experience, I've found that limiting food intake on the day prior to travel can help on a long-haul flight simply because it minimizes the feelings of bloatedness that can occur in the low cabin pressure of an airplane.

easily when the local time for sleep comes and you'll sleep for your normal number of hours (possibly a little bit more), waking at local morningtime. Within a couple of days, you should have reset your biological clock to the new time.

However, adjusting to eastward travel – speeding up the clock to reset it forward in time – tends to be more difficult. The timing of your light exposure is the key. There are excellent online jet lag calculators (see Resources, p.208) to help you work out when you need to expose yourself to light, but as a rule of thumb:

• Decide the time at which you usually wake up.

• Subtract two hours from that time to get a "start time".

• In your new destination, find light from that start time for at least two hours. (To slow down the clock, you should get light exposure for two hours *up to* the start time.) Over three to four days you should synchronize with local time, but it can take up to a fortnight, depending upon your age (the older you are, the harder the adjustment) and your biological-clock sensitivity.

Five ways to get into the zone

In addition to light therapy, the following are my top five tips for helping you to adjust to a new time zone.

- Avoid taking sleeping pills to help you sleep during your flight. Sleeping pills prevent you from reacting quickly in an emergency, and they can also cause you to stay still in your seat for too long, increasing your susceptibility to deep vein thrombosis. However, you may want to consider melatonin supplements, which are available over the counter in the USA and by prescription in the UK (see box, p.116).
- Take your meals according to the new time zone rather than the old one, as this helps to reset the circadian clock that governs your digestion. Mealtime synchronization is not a magic cure for jet lag, but it can have a knock-on effect that helps your sleep–wake cycle to readjust, too.
- At your destination, get up and do some light exercise in the morning, preferably in the open air. This will expose your body to natural light at the right time for waking, as well as giving your body a burst of energy and feel-good hormones that can set you up to feel positive and alert for the day.
- At your destination, structure your activities to take into account your body's existing circadian rhythm. For example, don't drive long distances during times when your body thinks it's nighttime, particularly between the hours of 2am and 6am at your home time zone.
- Break the normal rules and use caffeine to see you through patches of sleepiness, as long as they don't occur too close to the time when you do want to sleep.
- Some people find it helpful to set their watches to the new time zone as soon as they get on the airplane. This is fine, but beware if you take timed medication – make sure that you

SLEEP SCIENCE

MELATONIN – TIME ZONE TREATMENT

If you've ever seen a pharmacist or a doctor about overcoming jet lag (or dealing with shift work sleep problems), you may have been told about melatonin supplementation.

Secreted by the brain's pineal gland, melatonin is the hormone that responds to light and dark, telling you when to sleep and when to wake up. Taken as a supplement, it acts as a chronobiotic – which means it can alter the "time" of the biological clock and in doing so help you to cope with jet lag (or shift work). Most supplements are formulated to release melatonin much more quickly than we'd ever expect when the body secretes it naturally.

Different countries have different rules for the use of melatonin as a sleep-aid supplement. For example, in the UK supplements are available only by prescription issued by a medical practitioner; in the USA, they're available over the counter. Either way, as a rule, 1mg taken when you go to bed in the new time zone for up to three nights is sufficient to adjust to the new zone.

don't miss a dosage or, just as importantly, that you don't take too many dosages. If you do change your watch, keep something else (such as your cell phone) on home time, so that you have a point of reference for your medication.

Fatigue

Long-distance travel involves not only the time you're actually on the plane travelling (whether that's an 8- to 12-hour flight across one ocean, or 24 hours across several), but also the time it takes to get to the airport, check in, make your way through immigration, pick up your luggage, re-check it for very long journeys, collect it again and eventually head to your accommodation. It's hardly surprising that fatigue is an issue for long-distance travellers.

The best thing you can do for your body in order to minimize fatigue is to try to clock up some extra sleep one or two nights before your journey begins. Think of this as charging up your "sleep battery".

Once you're on your way, work out when your normal sleeping hours would be if you were still at home, and aim to get some sleep on the plane during those hours. In my experience, sleeping on the plane according to your home time zone does not hamper readjustment to the new time zone. In fact, you're more likely to adjust quickly if you don't feel fatigued. If your natural sleep time is during a period of activity for the aircraft crew, use an eye mask and ask the crew to leave you if you're sleeping when the food comes round.

Take something from home that you associate with falling sleep. For example, you could put a certain fragrance on your pillow for the nights running up to your trip. Lavender essence, which is claimed to have soporific qualities, is perfect. Take a handkerchief with that scent on the plane and put it where you can smell it as you try to sleep.

Stress

Many of my clients find travelling inherently stressful, which means that they are already set up for losing hours of sleep both in the nights before their journey and during the journey itself. In the week running up to your departure, try to practise this simple breathing meditation: close your eyes and visualize a square. As you breathe in, in your mind's eye you trace along the top of the square, and down one side as you breathe out. Breathe in again as you trace along the bottom of the square, and out again as you trace the line up to your starting corner. Based on a yoga breathing technique, this method is a quick-fix for when you need to relax on the plane and it's my favourite way to make sure I arrive at my destination feeling as fresh as possible. Practising it before you travel ensures your brain associates it with calming down.

AN ATHLETE'S GUIDE TO GOOD SLEEP

Whether you're a runner or a swimmer, a hurdler or a soccer player, all athletes (and sportspeople in general) need to sleep soundly if they are to gain the competitive edge in the sports arena. Sleep is essential for increased energy, performance and stamina, as well as improved alertness and mental agility. This is because:

- Sleep restores energy in our brain cells – mental energy becomes depleted over the course of the day as the mind processes information and directs the body in its daily tasks.
- Sleep can promote muscle growth and actively supports the mechanisms that store and restore energy in the muscles, in turn improving performance.
- Sleep helps to improve "muscle memory", a form of procedural memory (see pp.29–30) in which continued repetition of a certain muscle movement means that the movement becomes second nature – that is, the athlete can perform it without conscious effort (see box, opposite).
- Sleep maintains and improves waking mental processes.

One study at Stanford University in the USA has shown that athletes who increased their sleeping time from the normal seven to eight hours a night to between nine and ten hours, also significantly improved their speed and stamina in their sport.

Sleep time and performance

Elite performance demands the optimum in flexibility, strength, cardiovascular endurance, reaction time, memory, and attention. This means that during exercise both your muscle and your brain need to have a steady energy supply – which means a steady supply of glucose. Too few hours spent in good-quality sleep can have a dramatic impact on the body's metabolism, reducing its efficiency at converting glucose (sugars derived from carbohydrates) into usable energy by around a third. When your glucose reserves begin to run out, your body calls upon another carbohydrate called glycogen, which is mainly stored in your liver and fat cells and which provides an emergency source of energy during peak expenditure.

It's up to the hormone insulin, which regulates your metabolism and signals when your body needs to release energy stores, to make sure

MUSCLE MEMORY

Whatever sport you practise, you need to learn the movements – whether they're for jumping hurdles, kicking a ball or swinging a racquet. You need to hone your movements to respond quickly and accurately, perhaps even faster than your conscious processing allows. If you panic (in scientific terms, this means when your focused attention regresses to the point of almost forgetting what action you were supposed to take) or start to think too hard and lose automaticity (known as "choking"), your performance immediately deteriorates.

The fact that sleep improves muscle memory makes it an essential part of sports "training". Your body's memory of the movements you need for your sport is consolidated better when you're "offline". There are two reasons mooted for this. It could be that during sleep the consolidation of old or repeated memories is not subject to interference from ongoing (waking) activity. Or, it could be that during sleep your brain prunes down the action sequence to its greatest efficiency so that when you recall the action during practice, it's as honed as possible. Either way, through sleep your complex movements can become automatic, reducing incidence of panic and choking. All athletes aspiring to do their best need a good night's sleep.

that your glucose and glycogen levels meet your energy output. For some reason (we still don't know why), sleep deprivation interferes with your body's insulin signalling mechanism, which can result in inadequate supplies of glycogen when you need it. Quite simply, you start to run out of energy, a bit like a car running out of gas.

Training schedules place significant demands not only on the body but also on your time, with many athletes training early in the morning and late at night (this is particularly true of amateur athletes, who often have a day job to do in the meantime). The important thing is to try to make sure you get a good amount of good-quality sleep over the course of 24 hours – but how?

What you can do

- Set yourself a regular training/life schedule that you can follow every day, even at the weekends. Keeping to a regular routine helps to entrain your body so that it knows what to expect, including when to sleep. If you need to and can, consider having a siesta (see box, p.122). Establish a good pre-sleep routine (see pp.59–64) for this reason, too.
- It's better to do more training in the early morning (getting up early) so that you don't have to train later than 9pm in the evening. This should give your body enough time to settle down (including restoring normal body temperature) for a bedtime of 10pm, so that you're asleep by 10.30pm and can clock up eight hours sleep by 6.30am.
- Good athletes take rest days, but do try to get up and go to bed at the same time on your rest days as on your training days, so that you keep to your overall sleep–wake schedule.
- Read the advice for performers on pp.121–3 for tips on how to sleep after evening training sessions and how to time your siesta if you need one.

As with so many things to do with sleep, we're still exploring the precise relationship between sleep, performance and movement control. This makes it very hard to give definitive advice for athletes in general. It may be that your sport involves easily memorized sequences that don't require consolidation during sleep; or you may have no choice but to practise in the evening (and so need to find a sleep routine that allows you to get enough sleep). Use the advice that's applicable to you. In addition, consider whether or not you need to increase your sleeping hours in the run-up to a competition. Some athletes experience measurable improvements in their performance when they have a well-stocked sleep bank.

A PERFORMER'S GUIDE TO GOOD SLEEP

It might surprise some people to know that I'm not only a sleep expert, but also a dancer – although only in the amateur sense. I've found my feet in weekly sessions of the Argentine tango. However, if you're someone for whom performing – whether that's dancing, acting or singing, among others – is a job, a beloved hobby, or a way of life, special guidance can help you to get the best out of your sleep and also the best out of your performance.

Some individuals can perform in the evening, go home and fall quickly asleep, but this isn't the case for the majority. The physiological reasons you might find it hard to sleep after a performance are:

- Increased body temperature from sustained activity, which makes it harder to fall asleep.
- Increased levels of cortisol (the stress hormone), which is released naturally when we're doing something physically and emotionally demanding such as dancing, singing or acting.
- Increased levels of brain tryptophan and serotonin during activities that are physically and emotionally demanding, which cause initial feelings of fatigue, but then deplete, delaying sleep onset.
- Increased likelihood of phase delay – consistent late nights resulting in "owlish" tendencies.
- Use of caffeine supplements to enable prolonged periods of physical and mental activity.

Studies reveal that actors, dancers, musicians and even athletes who train during the evenings have a greater chance of turning to opiates, cigarettes, alcohol, recreational drugs and sleeping medication in order to wind down and get a good night's sleep. Such a lifestyle inevitably leads to casualties – including performers who have died as a result of addiction. Furthermore, performers for whom "ideal" body image is perceived as an essential part of the work have a greater chance of developing an eating disorder, such as bulimia or anorexia, not just because of how they look, but because a dysregulated metabolism (as a result of irregular cycles of wakefulness and sleep, activity and inactivity) causes bingeing or unhealthy eating and changes in appetite.

SLEEP THERAPY

MAKING UP THE DEFICIT

When you're performing, your schedule may make it impossible for you to get enough sleep during the hours of 11pm and 7am. You need to make up the deficit while keeping your internal clock set to the right social time as closely as possible.

1. Accept that you might need to keep a slightly unconventional daytime routine that includes a siesta. Do your best to keep to your sleep–wake routine even on your days off.
2. Take a nap in the early afternoon. Dim the lights, draw the blinds or curtains and get into bed. Sleep for between one and a half and two hours, which will give you enough time to have a whole cycle of sleep (see p.20). This nap will not only help you to repay the sleep debt, but also give you the stamina to provide a great performance later on. Make sure that you have 20 to 30 minutes to wake up fully before you have to go out.
3. Set your internal biological clock to the right social time by making sure that you face natural light, ideally bright sunlight, in the morning. Aim to get up at the same time every day, perhaps as early as 7.30am, but certainly not later than 8.30am.

What you can do

The key is to look at natural ways to optimize your sleep following a performance or evening rehearsal. Given that each of us is individual, what works for one may not work for others, so experiment with the guidelines below to identify what does work for you.

• Establish a pre-sleep ritual that helps to trigger your body and mind to understand that it's time for sleep. Follow this ritual every night – regardless of what time you get home. (Some or all of the following suggestions could form part of your ritual, if you like.)

- Before you go to bed, have a warm milky drink and a small piece of milk chocolate.
- Have a warm bath before you go to bed to relax your muscles, ease away any anxiety about your performance and gently relax following the adrenaline rush of being on stage; as well as to help to lower your body temperature.
- Keep your bedroom cool, and throw back your bedcovers in the morning so that your bed itself is cool when you get in.
- If you're using caffeine supplements to keep you energized, try to cut back on them and aim to take the last one no fewer than four hours before you intend to go to bed.
- Establish a daytime routine that you can stick to and that keeps your body clock on the right social time (see box, opposite).

A STUDENT'S GUIDE TO GOOD SLEEP

We already know that in sleep terms adolescence lasts from age 12 to about age 25, which for many people coincides with the years of being a student. Before we look at the specific sleep issues affecting students and how to overcome them, it's good to recap on the particular sleep–wake problems facing this age-group in general.

- The adolescent body clock operates more slowly than the true circadian rhythm (a condition known as phase delay), meaning that young people tend to have late nights and would naturally sleep later as a result.
- Adolescents have increased commitments to after-school clubs or extra-curricular activities that don't affect younger children, or even older adults, keeping them out later at night; they also inevitably have a time-consuming academic workload, particularly in the run-up to exams.
- Young people discover a burgeoning social life, which pulls them in a completely new direction that has to be slotted in with existing work and extra-curricular commitments.

All in all, the student years conspire to hamper good-quality sleep.

Student life

One study showed that only around ten percent of students at one university felt that they had a good night's sleep – which means falling asleep easily, sleeping undisturbed and waking up feeling refreshed.

In order for a student to perform to the best of his or her ability, he or she needs to be alert, focused, and composed under pressure. Only then can the brain become the perfect sponge for taking in new information, assimilating and storing it effectively and then recalling it accurately on demand. A good night's sleep is essential for all those processes to take place, so students need to do their best to work around the changing sleep patterns that go hand in hand with adolescence.

What you can do

If you're a school student living at home, it's important that you involve your parents in getting your sleep schedule right for your age and commitments. Talk through the following points with them and agree something that suits both of you – that way you'll reduce the risk of argument about whether or not you're getting enough sleep and you'll both know what you're aiming for.

If you're a college student, living on campus or in rented student accommodation, you'll be surrounded by temptation – parties, alcohol, recreational drugs – but you need to take responsibility for yourself, and that includes your commitment to your education, as well as to your health, well-being and lifestyle.

- Set a sleep schedule that you can stick to – having a routine is essential for making sure your body knows when it's time for sleep and when you need to be awake and alert. Use the guidelines in the box on page 126 to help you.
- Don't eat less than four hours before you go to bed, and if you attend an evening sports club try to make sure you have a good four hours between exercising and bedtime.
- Most students in college accommodation, and even students at school living at home, have a computer in their bedroom for study. Shut it down at least one hour before you go to bed. Your eyes (and brain) need time to rest before sleep.

- Don't use caffeine to keep you awake to make a deadline. If you feel sleepy – go to sleep! You'll work more effectively the following day, even if you have to get up early to finish off in time. Caffeine less than six hours before bedtime may disrupt your sleep if you're caffeine-sensitive (see pp.67–8).
- For those students of legal drinking age in the country in which you live, avoid alcohol altogether, or keep it to a minimum or for occasional dedicated nights out only. No one wants to be a party-pooper, but alcohol is a considerable sleep thief and will not help you with your studies!

Sleep and study assessment

In one survey at the University of San Diego, USA, almost 24 percent of college students believed that they had dropped grades in projects or examinations they'd undertaken at times when they felt particularly tired. That's almost a quarter of that year's college students who believed they could have done better. The problems they had may have ranged from misunderstanding questions to being unable to concentrate and (most crippling of all) "forgetting" everything they thought they'd learned. Elsewhere, I've known of students who've fallen asleep during an examination!

Playing hard and then cramming in the academic bits is not the way to sail through college. Instead, it's much better to pace yourself.

Both deep sleep and dreaming sleep enhance memory performance. However, if you've left the learning to the last minute with only a small window of opportunity to revise everything you need to know, try to stick to the following rough-and-ready rules.

- You'll remember better the information you learn between one and six hours before you go to sleep than what you learn outside the six-hour time window and under an hour before bed.
- Stop learning one hour before you intend to go to bed, so that you have time to wind down and so that learning can reach your hippocampus ready for consolidation (see p.29).
- Set an alarm to wake you at your normal waking time in the morning, so that you don't worry about oversleeping.

SLEEP THERAPY

MAPPING OUT YOUR STUDENT ROUTINE

So, you want to party, but you also know that it's important to get the most out of your education. Follow these steps to try to find a balance that permits the best of both worlds.

1. Make a list of the activities you're committed to (such as sports teams, any clubs, or a part-time job) and the times they occur. Taking the schedule as a whole, work out a time for bed – set a time that you can achieve to within half an hour every night.
2. Work out what time you need to get up in the morning in order to give yourself enough time to have breakfast, prepare for the day, and make it to school or college in good time.
3. If your allotted bedtime and rising time give you fewer than nine to ten hours sleep a night (see p.81), consider what commitments you could scale back on. Remember that your sleep is essential to your overall performance in academia – it's worth setting good sleep habits now to maximize what you get out of your education, and then later out of your adult life.
4. Once you've identified a routine that fits in with your lifestyle, try to be as strict as you can about sticking with that schedule. That's not to say that you shouldn't have any fun. If you're out at a party and get in late occasionally, that's fine – but make sure you get up at the usual time the following morning, making up the sleep debt by going to bed a little earlier the following night if necessary.

• It will take you at least 30 minutes to overcome "sleep inertia" – the fuggy period that occurs just after you wake up. On a revision day don't think about getting out of bed to begin cramming straightaway. Have a shower and breakfast before you sit down to the first period of study for the day.

• Take regular breaks during your revision (every two hours or so) and if you feel sleepy allow yourself a 30-minute nap. Many students find that a good pattern is to learn in the morning, then have lunch, a nap and another period of study, and then to stop at least an hour before bedtime so that they have a good night's sleep and are set up for more learning the following day.

A PARENTS' GUIDE TO GOOD SLEEP

This section is not about setting sleep routines for your newborn – all that is covered on pages 74–81. Rather, this is an area reserved for parents, an essential survival guide that helps you gain back the lost hours of nighttime sleep that inevitably come with a new baby. And not just with a new baby, with a toddler, and even a teenager, too.

A new baby's erratic and broken sleeping patterns can last for the first two years of life – and sometimes beyond. For parents this is a difficult time of juggling their own sleep needs and their ability to function during the day, with their instinct for nurturing, soothing and comforting their babies. In all likelihood, it's a time of limited sleep.

Whether or not a baby sleeps well doesn't seem to be an inherited trait. Even if you, your partner and all your family always slept well, your baby may well be the exception. Either way, your baby's sleep affects you. Sadly, there's no definitive research to tell you the best way to handle your child's sleeping so that you get the most out of your own sleep, especially as so much depends on cultural expectations of childhood sleep. For example, in Italy and Japan it's common to allow children into the parent's bedroom (where they might disturb you more often). In warmer climes, children may take a siesta and then stay up far later into the night. All you can do is take some advice and work out what works best for you and for your child.

What you can do
The baby years
Babies represent an "emergency situation" for parents. Babies' sleep schedules involve a lot of nighttime awakenings for food and comfort.

Conventionally, the advice has always been that in order to make up the lost hours of sleep, mothers (and fathers) should nap during the day. In 2010, research published by West Virginia University in the USA revealed that mothers who follow this guideline do appear to get enough hours asleep, but the poor quality of that sleep means that they still feel unrefreshed. The research likened the sleep of a new mother to someone with sleep apnoea – frequent awakenings, some of them barely perceptible, but amounting to broken sleep cycles and so non-restorative sleep. On top of that, on average mothers were awake for up to two hours a night for feeding and comforting. We know that mothers who rack up a large sleep debt are more likely to suffer post-natal depression, so it's essential to find ways to halt the trend.

To get through this difficult time (and it's worth remembering that these early months of sleep debt will pass), both parents need to share the workload as much as possible, both of you getting as much sleep as you can (see also the box, opposite). Don't worry about the washing, the dishes, the cleaning; and ignore the sleep-hygiene rules about daytime napping – do take naps and make them as long as you can. If you can nap for two hours, you can clock up at least one complete sleep cycle, and in this way wake feeling more refreshed. As far as is practicable, if one of you is napping and the baby wakes, the other can take charge. Most babies can go for a couple of hours between feeds, so in the early days even breastfeeding mums can get long naps if someone is on hand to help to take care of the baby.

As your baby gets slightly older (say, between 3 and 12 months), and into more of a routine, try to "anchor" your own sleep at certain times of day. That is, even if you aren't getting a full night, try to nap at the same times every day, aiming for 90 minutes to two hours each time. Above all, don't resort to sleep aids or alcohol, which dull your senses and reduce your sensitivity to your baby's needs.

The toddler years

The period from babyhood to toddlerhood is time to start introducing the principles of sleep hygiene to your child and to reinstate those principles in your own life, too. Once your baby understands about

SLEEP CLINIC

I want to help at night with our new baby, but I have to go to work in the morning. I feel guilty. What can I do?

Many companies are sympathetic to the demands of new parenthood, but if your company can't offer you a place to have a lunchtime nap, the easiest way round your problem is to set an agenda at home to cover the nightshifts that have the least impact for you at work and on other days for you to make an active contribution to running the household.

During the week the majority of the sleep bank goes to you; but for one night in the week if you can, and certainly at the weekends, you swap roles. This means that for three nights out of seven (say, Friday, Saturday and Sunday; or Thursday, Friday and Saturday), you deal with the baby's nighttime waking. If your partner is breastfeeding, perhaps she could express the feeds for your nights so that she can get the most out of her nights off.

During the week, pick up the groceries on the way home, make simple suppers and put on the odd load of laundry so that your partner doesn't feel that he or she needs to run the household alone, as well as to look after the baby. Sometimes just knowing that you don't mind coming home to dirty dishes is enough.

At the weekends or on your days off, revel in some extra baby-time, so that your partner can catch up on some sleep. (Incidentally, this rest should be in bed and far away from chores.) This is a great time for you to bond with the baby, as well as to help your partner.

If you both need to catch up on some sleep at the weekends, don't be afraid to ask for help from family or close friends you can trust. Most babies have an army of willing relatives who will relish some time to get to know the family's newest member. Don't be embarrassed to capitalize on that. Well-rested parents are happy parents, and that means that the baby's happy, too.

the long sleep through the night, your own sleep should begin to take a turn for the better. Nonetheless, children often have nightmares or night terrors and they are far more susceptible than adults many other parasomnias (see pp.156–65). Comforting your child during the night means that your own sleep is disturbed, and the only way to balance this is to keep napping during the day if you need to. Time your nap for early afternoon, though, and if you have a pre-school age child, encourage him or her to nap then, too. At the very least, both of you should have an hour of quiet, calm activity, sharing a book or doing a puzzle or even watching a little TV together.

The teenage years

Just as parents get used to their children sleeping more soundly, come the teenage years. The chances are you're likely to get plenty of sleep yourself (except on the nights when you have to pick up from a late party), and the problems are more likely to shift to managing your teenager's sleep. See pages 81–5 for advice.

A DREAMER'S GUIDE TO GOOD SLEEP

Jim Horne, Emeritus Professor of Psychophysiology at Loughborough University in the UK, once described dreaming as our own personal cinema. However, unlike a movie, dreams are not necessarily of our choosing. Nightmares aside, some people suffer from a disorder called "epic dreaming" in which dreams become kaleidoscopic, rollercoaster journeys that appear to last all night, apparently leaving the dreamer exhausted. Others claim to have no dreams at all.

I've never been fascinated by the interpretation of dreams. To me, when I consider the literature, dream interpretation tends to be specific to a particular society or culture, even though some psychoanalysts, such as Carl Jung (1875–1961), did explore the possibility of universal "archetypes" – symbols that are common to us all. My interest in dreams lies more in trying to understand their lucidity (our awareness of them; see box, p.23). Lucid dreams become really interesting when you can start to control them – we can have unlimited adventures, and

SLEEP CLINIC

Will cheese help me to dream?

While I haven't been able to find any scientific evidence that cheese promotes dreams, many people do say that a good, ripe blue cheese will do the trick – but the evidence is anecdotal. On the other hand, a study in 2002 revealed tentative findings that vitamin B6 supplements might indeed promote more vivid dreams. You can find B6 in such foods as avocados, brewer's yeast, broad beans, bananas, molasses, salmon and herring. A warm cup of milk spiced with a little nutmeg two to three hours before you go to bed is also supposed to work.

safe rehearsal time to deal with nightmares or traumatic events; lucid dreams can even help with problem-solving (see pp.135–6).

Recognizing and remembering your dreams

In Chapter 2 we looked at the science of dreaming – the neurological processes that go on in our brains in order for dreams to happen. Here, we're going to take that science and apply it to the activity of dreaming, so that we can learn to dream lucidly.

Throughout this book I've talked about how various brain states that involve parts of the brain either shutting down or switching on. Both sleep and wakefulness are highly synchronized states. If that synchrony fails, new states arise – one of which is dreaming (this is why dreaming sleep is sometimes referred to as "paradoxical sleep" – we have an active, but sleeping brain while our muscles are paralyzed). In dreams we perceive what's going on in our brains while we're in the dreaming (R) stage of sleep, and occasionally in other sleep stages, too. Sleep paralysis, out-of-body experiences and hypnagogic hallucinations are other examples of a lack of synchrony.

The first thing to say is that we're all capable of dreaming. We go into dreaming sleep roughly every 90 minutes and we tend to have

THE APP OF DREAMS

Modern technology has provided us with many new ways to understand from our own beds the nature of sleep. Smartphone app technology enables you to place your phone on your bed and use it to influence your dreams. Certain apps will detect when you enter dreaming sleep and then play pre-recorded sounds of the sorts of landscapes or scenarios you want to enter in your dreams. For example, if you tell the app you want to dream about being by the sea, it will play seascape sounds as you enter dreaming sleep. See the Resources on page 208 for information on how to find the app.

longer periods of it toward the end of the night. This happens for everyone. Recalling our dreams usually occurs when we wake shortly after, or even during, a period of R sleep. Those people who think they don't dream, probably do – it's just that by the time they wake, their last period of dreaming sleep is too far from consciousness for them to remember what they dreamed about.

So, before we can learn to control our dreams, we have to learn to notice and to remember them. You could get quite sophisticated and use a sleep gadget (such as a Zeo; see box, p.202) to alert you with a soft tone when you enter R. However, you can also simply go to bed with the positive conviction that you'll connect with your dreams when they happen. Furthermore, since ancient times people have been developing methods of "dream incubation" – sowing the seeds of a dream during waking hours and directing their minds to attend to whatever is going on in it. In this simple technique all you have to do is spend a few minutes contemplating the subject of your dream before you go to bed and tell yourself that you'll recall your dreams when you wake. I've set out the method in the box on page 134.

I recommend that you keep a dream journal. The more you make a point of recalling the details of your dreams (whether you incubated them or not), the more attentive you'll become to them, and this forms the beginnings of lucid dreaming. Keep a notebook and pen beside your bed. If you wake up in the night from a dream and want to note it down, you can do so (while the details are fresh). Otherwise, write down what you can recall in the morning. Don't try to edit your notes – allow the dream visions to come back to you in the same fragmented ways that they appeared. You aren't necessarily trying to make sense of what you dreamed about, merely to recall as much detail as possible so that your dreams start to gain your full, sleeping attention.

Achieving lucidity

Research is still not entirely clear as to what technique is best to achieve lucidity, but there are two main approaches that appear to work. The first is the mental or cognitive approach and the second is through physical stimulation. In general, though, both these rely on some work while you're awake to prepare you for lucid dreaming.

There are two cognitive approaches that appear to work best to promote lucid dreaming. Using either of these, or combining them, along with using physical techniques provides the best basis for lucidity.

Tholey's method

The German psychologist Paul Tholey (1937–1998) developed the "reflection technique". During the day ask yourself at several points, "Am I awake, or am I dreaming?" and consciously work out how you know you're awake. Then you imagine what your surroundings would be like if you were in a dream. In these ways you become more attuned to the differences between wakefulness and dreaming, so that you can learn to recognize your dreaming state more easily when it happens. As you fall asleep you repeatedly tell yourself, "I am going to lucid-dream." The combination of reflection and auto-suggestion enables you to put yourself in your dreams and to begin controlling them.

LaBerge's method

The American psychophysiologist Stephen LaBerge has developed a technique he calls MILD – Mnemonic Induction of Lucid Dreams.

SLEEP THERAPY

INCUBATING YOUR DREAMS

You can use the following exercise as a pre-sleep relaxation in place of any other you already perform (if you do). I suggest you sit comfortably on your bed or on your bedroom floor.

1. Sit in a balanced position with your back straight and your shoulders relaxed. Breathe deeply for a few minutes.

2. Bring to mind the topic or scenario you want to dream about. You're going to turn it into a creative visualization – imagining it in as much detail as possible. For example, if you want to dream about being on vacation, call up the landscape in fine detail; imagine yourself in the scene – swimming in the ocean, horseback riding through the forest, hiking along mountain paths. Who is with you? What are you wearing? What's the weather like? What can you hear, smell, see?

3. Spend ten minutes in quiet reflection on your dream scenario. Then, repeat to yourself five times, slowly and softly: "I will dream. I will remember my dreams." Now you're ready to go to bed. (In the morning, compare your dream scenario to the one you'd imagined. What fantastical elements did your unconscious create that your conscious imagination did not?)

Involving a fair amount of preparatory work, MILD requires you first hone your waking observation and memory. LaBerge recommends taking four target occurrences from the day, and making a point of noticing when these occur. For example, you might choose a dog barking, turning right, seeing a flower, and seeing your face in the mirror. Each time you encounter one of these targets in a day, you make a conscious note that it's happened. Every day you choose four new targets and you practise the method for a week, after which time hopefully you'll find yourself competent enough to use your entry into a dream as a target to achieve lucidity. In a way that is similar to Tholey's method, you go to bed resolving that you'll be lucid during your dreams and that you'll recall your dreams in the morning. Tell yourself, "Next time I dream, I want to remember I'm dreaming."

Physical methods

Methods that involve light, acoustic or tactile stimuli to alert you to the fact that you're entering dreaming sleep used to be the province of the sleep laboratory, but there are now several gadgets and gizmos (including the Zeo; see box, p.202) that you can buy to use at home. You have to go to bed telling yourself that once you realize a light is flashing, or you hear a particular sound or feel a particular sensation (the trigger will depend upon which gadget you're using), you'll know you're in R sleep and therefore dreaming.

For all the methods, you have to go bed with a detached and neutral mind, so that you don't get too excited when you realize you're in dreaming sleep and wake yourself up! Once you notice you're dreaming, you can start trying to manipulate your dream. You can try to fly, walk on water, achieve superhuman feats, vanquish monsters, practise your dance moves, or overcome issues from the day ... whatever you like.

A PROBLEM-SOLVER'S GUIDE TO GOOD SLEEP

From Albert Einstein to Paul McCartney and from Samuel Taylor Coleridge to Jack Nicklaus, the great, the good and the utterly brilliant have claimed flashes of inspiration and creativity during their sleep. In the case of Einstein, it's said that he germinated the Theory of Relativity when he dreamed of sledging down a mountainside and noticing how the appearance of the stars changed relative to his speed. Paul McCartney is said to have written the tune for "Yesterday" in a dream; Coleridge dreamed his poem *Kubla Khan*; and Jack Nicklaus dreamed up a new grip for golf clubs. Whatever the problem, it seems that our sleep, and our dreams, may have the answer.

Most of us know the experience of "sleeping on it" – leaving a problem unresolved only to experience a "eureka!" moment (or, indeed, the slow advancement to a solution) during the night. Sleep does more than just allow the passage of resting time. It reduces the interference of daytime activity so that there are fewer distractions, and fewer mounting problems to deal with or responses to give, permitting the problem-solving parts of the brain to work undisturbed.

Previously I've described how different stages of sleep have different effects on different types of memory; and memory experiments have shown that the way individual memories relate to each other (associate) actively changes during sleep – all of which facilitates problem solving. Furthermore, tentative studies in the USA have shown that, following periods of dreaming sleep, subjects are better able to find solutions to creative tasks. During sleep, and particularly during R, the brain seems better able to make new pathways (associations) between pieces of data, and so finds more efficient routes to the answer to a problem. In one experiment, researchers asked participants to work out the next numbers in a sequence. Subjects were given a lengthy method for finding the answers, which they used perfectly successfully. Then, some participants were asked to sleep and others merely to rest. On repeating the task, those who'd slept were more likely to have found a hidden shortcut to the answers, while the resters mostly continued to use the long method they'd been taught in the first place. It appears that during sleep the brain had had a "eureka!" moment, working out the quickest route to resolution.

Now it's your turn

It's all very well that the brain can randomly solve a problem that it encounters during the day, but is it possible to "ask" it to tackle something specific? One method would be to use lucid dreaming – I've described in detail on pages 133–5 how to begin to control your dreams and there's no reason why you can't adapt the techniques given there to include musing on a particular problem. Alternatively, you can simply hold your problem in your mind as you fall asleep, in the hope that as it was the last thing you thought about, your brain will take the problem and run with it, creating pathways that can take you to the answer when you wake.

CHAPTER 6

SLEEP DISORDERS –
STEP BY STEP

Since writing my first book on insomnia many years ago, there have been considerable developments in our understanding of sleep – and that inevitably means that we've learned a lot about insomnia, too. Over the following pages I shall introduce you to all the major sleep disorders, several different insomnias among them, tell you what characterizes them and give you tips on how to overcome them. A simple "Insomnia Matrix" helps you to unravel your symptoms to work out which disorders might apply to you.

Throughout the chapter it's important to bear in mind that many sleep disorders can become or are from the outset serious conditions and you may need to seek individualized professional advice. If you're at all worried, see your medical practitioner and, if necessary, ask for a referral to a sleep specialist. Almost all sleep disorders are perfectly treatable as long as you have the right level of support.

SLEEP DISORDERS CLASSIFIED

At the last count, the International Classification of Sleep Disorders listed 81 conditions that affect the quality of our sleep. Although this number is high, in effect the conditions fall into only eight categories:

1. Insomnias
2. Hypersomnias, including narcolepsy
3. Parasomnias
4. Circadian Rhythm Sleep Disorders
5. Sleep-related Breathing Disorders
6. Sleep-related Movement Disorders
7. Isolated Symptoms, Apparently Normal Variants and Unresolved Issues (basically the sleep-disorder loose ends)
8. Sleep Disorders Associated with Conditions Classifiable Elsewhere, of which there are 14 different conditions. These include sleep-related epilepsy, headaches, gastroesophageal reflux disease (such as heartburn), coronary artery ischemia (heart problems), abnormal swallowing, choking, and laryngospasm, as well as mental disorders that cause sleep problems, including depression, anxiety and schizophrenia. Sufferers in this group must tackle the physical or psychological issues at the root of their sleep problem, in the hope that better sleep will follow (adding good sleep hygiene can only help the situation, too).

It would take a volume of books to cover all the sleep disorders in all the categories in full, so over the following pages I've selected the major insomnias and sleep disorders for special treatment. I explain what each is, what causes each, and provide ideas on how to improve your sleep if you think one of them is affecting you. I've also presented some of the more unusual disorders – to illustrate just how diverse and how extraordinary your sleep is or can be.

At several points in this chapter, I've suggested that you keep a sleep diary for two weeks in order to better understand your sleep problems and symptoms. There are some disorders for which it is especially useful to have a record of your sleep, but a sleep diary can help whatever you think the problem is. Use the template on pages 140–141 as a starting point, and add any columns you think you might need. For example, you might want to add a column in which to note whether or not you remember dreaming that night; or whether or not you experienced a recurring sleep disorder.

Sleep diary template You can copy out the template by hand or reproduce it from here if you like. Keep the diary for two weeks in order to get a full picture of your sleeping and waking habits.

Filling in the grid
- Put a U in the box at the time at which you get out of bed.
- Put an S in the box that represents any time when you feel sleepy during the day (but did not actually nap).
- Put a heart in the box to show time you spend exercising.
- Put a dot in the box to indicate when you have any caffeine.
- Put a circle in the box when you have an alcoholic drink.
- Put a + in the box when you take any medication.
- Shade in any hours in which you take a daytime nap.
- Put a tick in the box when you go to bed.
- Put an R in the box for time you're reading in bed.
- Put an F in the box at the time you estimate you fell asleep, and a W for the time you wake up. Use a solid line to indicate the hours of tranquil sleep and a wobbly line for broken sleep.

INSOMNIA: AN OVERVIEW
Insomnia is an umbrella term for several different conditions, all of them serious. These conditions are different from sleeplessness in that they develop over time, prevent you from sleeping when you want to sleep and affect how you function during the day. Insomnia might have developed as a secondary condition (that is, triggered by something else), or it might be "comorbid" – that is, it may occur at the same time as another condition, but not because of it. Characteristically, though, insomnia has no obvious cause at all.

The American Academy of Sleep Medicine has identified several different types of insomnia: I've covered the main ones over the following pages. Broadly, however, insomnia is pigeon-holed by the length of time it's been going on (whether it's acute or chronic) and by its sub-type (whether it occurs "early", "mid" or "late" into the night).

In recent years, researchers have tried to identify how each type

Day	Date	Work/Day off/School	9 am	10 am	11 am	Mid-day	1 pm	2 pm	3 pm	4 pm	5 pm
Saturday											
Sunday											
Monday											
Tuesday											
Wednesday											
Thursday											
Friday											
Saturday											
Sunday											
Monday											
Tuesday											
Wednesday											
Thursday											
Friday											

6 pm	7 pm	8 pm	9 pm	10 pm	11 pm	Mid-night	1 am	2 am	3 am	4 am	5 am	6 am	7 am	8 am

of insomnia develops, building up several layers of explanation. The explanations all begin with the simple idea that most insomnia is caused by hyperarousal, a state in which a person's brain is simply too excited to sleep. In order for us to fall asleep, the brain has to go into a state of "de-arousal" or "sub-arousal". If the normal processes that make that happen don't work (in particular, if the brain can't switch off from the "fight or flight" response), a state of hyperarousal can occur. We can be certain that hyperarousal is a problem for sleep health because medicines that reduce arousal – known as tranquillizers – and help to switch off the brain also help people to get to sleep.

Hyperarousal has several different psychological models, but fundamentally if you have insomnia, you'll fulfil the following conditions:
• You find it hard to fall asleep or to stay asleep.
• You can find no obvious cause why you can't sleep.
• You have impaired ability to function in your waking hours.

All the sections in this chapter deal with a specific type of insomnia, or a sleep disorder. In order that you can establish which of these sleep thieves might apply to you, I've created an Insomnia Matrix that asks broad questions about your sleep and wakefulness so that you can go on to read the advice most relevant to your situation.

The Insomnia Matrix

The Matrix on pages 144–5 is designed to help you decide whether or not you have an insomnia or another type of sleep disorder. In many cases your symptoms could result from several different disorders, some of which may occur as a result of or in addition to a general insomnia. Take time to look at the Matrix and establish which disorders could be affecting you, then read the relevant pages for more information and tips on how to improve your sleeping life.

The Matrix assumes that you have already established good levels of sleep hygiene (see Chapter 3), but that even optimizing every aspect of your sleep hygiene hasn't resulted in any improvement in your sleep. Remember that insomnia is the result of chronic sleeplessness without known cause. If you know why you aren't sleeping soundly, you have a sleep disorder (not insomnia) or other condition that's affecting your sleep. Dealing with that will therefore inevitably help you to sleep more soundly. And, finally, there are many reasons other than a sleep disorder that may lead to tiredness – refer back to the boxes on pages 6–7 to make sure that none of those apply, too.

Using the matrix

Look at the column on the far left and find the statements that apply to you (some you'll know are true only because your bed partner has told you so), then look across the matrix to see which sleep disorders or insomnias each statement may signify (denoted by a star). Make a note of the possibilities and then read those sections on the following pages for more information and advice. Bear in mind that it's possible you have more than one disorder.

ADJUSTMENT INSOMNIA

According to the definition set by the International Classification of Sleep Disorders, you have adjustment (or acute) insomnia when you aren't able to sleep when you want to, but know (or are fairly certain you know) why it is that sleep won't come – that is, you know what's stressing you out. For me, this is rather more like sleeplessness because, by definition, true insomnia has no known cause.

Causes

Studies indicate that adjustment insomnia affects between 15 and 20 percent of adults every year. I think almost everyone is susceptible, although some are more susceptible than others. If you've had periods of anxiety or depression in the past, are prone to living by your emotions (good and bad), and find it especially hard to deal with stress, or unwind or relax, you may be more likely to suffer from this.

Moving to a new home and finding it hard to get used to, a personal loss, diagnosis of a medical condition, relationship problems, troublesome work colleagues or superiors, ongoing arguments with authority, as well as intense happiness, love or infatuation can all cause adjust-

	Insomnias	Hypersomnias (including narcolepsy)	Parasomnias (including night terrors and sleepwalking)	Circadian rhythm disorders	Sleep-related breathing disorders (including snoring and sleep apnoea)	Sleep-related movement disorders (including restless leg syndrome)	Disorders known as "Normal variants"	Mental disorders
I have high blood pressure					✸			
I am gaining weight	✸				✸			
I have fallen asleep when laughing or crying		✸						
I feel like someone is in the room with me (but isn't)			✸					
I feel like I am hallucinating when I fall asleep		✸	✸					✸
I have vivid dreams soon after falling asleep		✸						✸
I experience aching or "crawling" sensations in my legs						✸		
I jerk my legs before I fall asleep, sometimes violently						✸	✸	

Statement							
I thrash or kick out during my sleep			✶	✶			
I have trouble falling asleep					✶		
I talk in my sleep		✶				✶	
I wake up in the night and can't go back to sleep					✶		
I seem to feel tired all day			✶	✶			
I snore, gasp for air, or pant in my sleep		✶		✶			
I often need the loo in the night, several times a night				✶		✶	
I feel like I'm hallucinating almost all night							✶
I have nightmares	✶					✶	
I often doze off during the day				✶		✶	✶
I wake up and I can't move		✶				✶	

ment insomnia. You may find that your nighttime insomnia has a daytime counterpart in ruminative thoughts or worries, or an inability to focus on anything other than your anxiety or indeed elation.

Treatments

On the whole, adjustment insomnia disappears, and normal sleeping patterns resume, once you've dealt with the stressor, or have adapted to your new situation. In insomnia terms, you're very lucky, because you know what the root cause of your problem is.

Importantly, try not to resort to artificial methods to improve your sleep. Alcohol, recreational drugs, so-called sleep medicines and even natural remedies for sleep do not tackle the root cause of adjustment insomnia. If it's simply a matter of time to get used to living in a new house, functioning in a new environment and so on, speed up the process by making your new environment a more comfortable place to be. In a new home, hold a housewarming party, redecorate to your taste, and so on. In a new job, arrange a social gathering with your new colleagues so that you more quickly feel part of the team. If personal matters, such as a relationship problem, personal loss, or bereavement, are causing your anxiety, seek specialist advice or counselling so that by dealing with your emotions you tackle your insomnia.

A word of warning: don't let adjustment insomnia rattle on in the hope that it will cure itself. Although it is by definition a temporary condition, adjustment insomnia can herald the beginning of something more persistent. If your stressor causes your body to react with the "fight or flight" response – that is, an adrenaline surge that results in increased heart-rate, breathing, sweating, and so on – and you don't find effective ways to overcome that stress, normalize your adrenaline levels and establish a sense of equilibrium again, you may become preoccupied with your inability to sleep. In turn, sleep may become something that you feel you have to work at, rather than something that comes naturally when you feel sleepy. The result can be psychophysiological insomnia, the most common form of persistent insomnia, which I explain next. (Also, don't forget good sleep hygiene!)

SLEEP THERAPY

IDENTIFYING STRESS-RELATED SLEEPLESSNESS

Disturbed sleep often arises from stress. You can check whether or not this is true for you by answering the questions below. The more "yes" answers you give, the more possible it is that stress is the primary cause of your sleeplessness. Take steps to reduce stress before establishing whether or not you also have a sleep disorder.

1. Have you experienced significant unintended weight gain or weight loss recently?
2. Are you putting weight on, particularly around your tummy?
3. Has your libido decreased, or are you too tired for sex?
4. Do you feel tense, especially in your neck, back and jaw?
5. Do you experience tension headaches?
6. Do you find that you're more sensitive, irritable or easily frustrated than you used to be?
7. Do you have a general feeling of being overwhelmed by everything you're dealing with right now?
8. Do you feel always overtired or exhausted?
9. Do you find it more difficult to make decisions and/or concentrate?
10. Do you forget things more often than you used to?
11. Do you find that you're ill more often than usual?
12. Do you often feel anxious about things you can't control?
13. Do you find yourself eating to cope with annoyances, or craving sweet or salty food?
14. Do you find yourself drinking alcohol to relax or smoking to deal with stress, or are you becoming dependent on illegal drugs or prescribed medication?

PSYCHOPHYSIOLOGICAL INSOMNIA

Also known as learned or conditioned insomnia, primary insomnia, chronic insomnia or the rather esoteric-sounding "functionally autonomous insomnia", psychophysiological insomnia is characterized by a racing mind that results from a combination of hyperarousal (when the body can't wind down from the stress response) and learned associations that prevent sleep occurring. Most often sufferers become overly concerned with falling asleep, which results in them remaining awake instead. Sufferers are unable to identify any particular stress or anxiety that might prevent them from sleeping, other than the need for sleep itself. It's thought that up to two percent of people in the UK and ten percent of people in the USA suffer from psychophysiological insomnia, and for reasons we don't fully understand it affects women more often than it affects men.

Compared with normal sleepers, psychophysiological insomniacs pay attention to their sleep, and by extension their sleeplessness and the effects of sleep loss. Good sleepers have minimal "intent to sleep" – in other words, they're more able to let go of wakefulness. A psychophysiological insomniac expends effort to find sleep; sleep is no longer the natural, automatic result of sleepiness but something that the sleeper has to work at.

Studies show that there are certain questions and anxieties that recur among insomniacs of this kind, including:

- Anxiety over the importance of sleep in order to function normally during the day. You might say such things as, "If I don't sleep, I won't be able to do all the work I have to do tomorrow," or "I'm tired and irritable because I can't sleep."
- Breaking down old associations, such as the bed being a place conducive to a good night's sleep, and replacing them with negative ones. You might say such things as "I can't get into a comfortable position", "I toss and turn because I'm so worked up that I'm in bed and not sleeping" and "I lie in bed trying harder and harder to fall asleep." Similar shifts in association might happen with a bedtime routine – once a precursor to sleep, the actions instead herald sleeplessness.

Causes

For many, although by no means all, psychophysiological insomnia begins as adjustment insomnia (see pp.143–6), when a stressful event may trigger a short period of insomnia that then leads to overanxiety about sleep and so to psychophysiological insomnia. For others, the worry about sleep develops slowly – even over months and years. Gradually sleep deteriorates until the goal of getting a "good night's sleep" becomes paramount and, by a cruel irony, unachievable.

Effects

Psychophysiological insomniacs suffer from fatigue, poor concentration and low mood, and general malaise. They find not only that nighttime sleep eludes them, but that daytime napping is impossible, too. In sleep centres, studies indicate that psychophysiological insomniacs have fewer hours of deep and dreaming sleep, reduced sleep efficiency and generally reduced numbers of hours asleep.

In the long term, the persistent lack of sleep and ongoing feelings of helplessness may all lead to clinical depression.

Treatments

Patients often tell me that they begin to sleep better from the moment they've made an appointment to see me. Others find that they get a good night's sleep when they spend a night in a sleep centre. These consequences tell me two things. First, that overcoming psychophysiological insomnia is partly a question of taking control of sleep, believing that sleep will come because something has changed (making an appointment, passing sleep concerns on to someone else to deal with) and, second, in part the insomnia is related to associations my patients make with their beds (in the sleep centre beds, they fall asleep).

The key then is to start unravelling the negative associations you have with your bed and bedroom, as well as those you may have with your sleep routine and even with sleep itself. Doing so takes time, but the following can help to ease the process.

• Redecorate your bedroom or move around the furniture in it.
  Declutter the space (nothing on top of wardrobes or stuffed

under beds) and treat yourself to some new bedding. This "new" space is one in which you'll sleep well. At an extreme, you could treat yourself to a new mattress (see pp.54–8) or bed so that you break the negative associations you hold with the one you already have. However, note that psychophysiological insomnia is primarily about reconditioning your mind – this should be your first objective, and it needn't be expensive.

- Change your bedtime routine. Although there are certain things that you have to do (locking the door, brushing your teeth and so on), try some alternative triggers as well. For example, if you're used to drinking a warm cup of milk before bed, switch to a cup of herbal (uncaffeinated) tea instead. Valerian root has been shown to have some soporific qualities (see box, p.201). If you've been practising progressive muscle relaxation before you get into bed (see box, p.63), try autogenic training instead (see pp.71–2).
- Spend 20 to 30 minutes outdoors doing light to moderate exercise every day, not less than four hours before you go to bed. This helps to raise your mood, making you feel more positive about sleep. It'll also release muscle tension so that discomfort doesn't exacerbate your inability to get to sleep.
- Consider Cognitive Behaviour Therapy for Insomnia – in which a therapist teaches you coping strategies for your existing thought processes, as well as strategies for re-convincing yourself that sleep is in fact a positive, accessible state, rather than the elusive one it has become. As a first step, you can try the Stimulus Control method (see box, opposite).

OTHER FORMS OF INSOMNIA

Whereas psychophysiological insomnia is a learned insomnia (that is, it occurs because of your own anxieties about sleep), the following insomnias may be acquired as a result of genetics (traits you've inherited from your ancestors) or as a result of a life event that has caused trauma.

SLEEP THERAPY

REMAKING ASSOCIATIONS

The following steps use "Stimulus Control" in which three simple instructions are designed to re-associate the bed and bedroom with sleep, and to help re-entrain your biological clock to the correct cycles of sleep and wakefulness. The method is very simple, and it works – so even though it might seem inflexible, stick with it and eventually you will see some results.

1. Go to bed only when you feel sleepy – not simply fatigued, but properly sleepy.
2. If after 20 minutes in bed you're unable to sleep, get out of bed, go to another room, sit quietly doing nothing (no reading and certainly no television), and return to bed only when you feel that you're about to fall asleep.
3. Use the bed and bedroom only for sleep.

Idiopathic insomnia

Also known as "childhood onset insomnia", idiopathic insomnia is one of the rarest forms of insomnia of all, affecting less than one percent of the general population. It usually appears from birth, with babies finding it hard to settle at night and yet appearing drowsy and unfocused during the day. Its root cause continues to baffle sleep scientists, and although research into twins has suggested that the condition may be inherited, we're still far from knowing for sure.

Investigations at sleep centres tentatively reveal that idiopathic insomniacs have trouble falling and staying asleep. Their sleep patterns show irregularities similar to those found in psychophysiological insomnia – fewer periods of deep sleep, disturbed sleep, frequent unexplained awakenings, and so on – but they tend to be more severe. Brain imaging studies show that areas that are usually less active during sleep are more active; while those that should be more active during wakefulness quieten down. The result is that at night the idiopathic insomniac can't sleep, while during the day he or she finds it hard to concentrate, and may suffer other cognitive problems. Because the condition tends to be present from very early on in a sufferer's life, most sufferers find ways to live with it – adapting their lifestyles so that they achieve enough sleep in each 24 hours to function properly.

This is a good thing, as sleep experts can't agree on the best way to treat the condition. Some find that Cognitive Behavioural Therapy for Insomnia might work (see box, p.197), but because the insomnia is not the result of stress, or negative associations, or even poor sleep hygiene, there doesn't seem to be a clear answer on what to do. Nonetheless, training the body to prepare for sleep, through establishing a clear and rigid sleep routine, is essential to minimizing the effects and ensuring that a night's sleep is as good as it can be.

Paradoxical insomnia

You'll almost certainly know how it feels to be unsure how long you've been awake during the night – although for sound sleepers any misperception is usually by only a few minutes. If you have paradoxical insomnia you'll feel you've slept for very few hours when in fact you've slept for many. The problem might occur when two short periods of wakefulness are perceived as a single, long block. The disorder tends to begin during early adulthood and occurs in both men and women.

Paradoxical insomnia is a "sleep state misperception". This form of insomnia became apparent only when sleep researchers started recording insomniacs. A small percentage were found to sleep for seven to eight hours a night despite reporting that they had slept for only one to two hours. However, their sleep was not refreshing.

Doctors once thought that sleeping pills were the only way to overcome this kind of insomnia. In fact, recent research shows that reducing the amount of time you spend in bed to just longer than the amount of time you perceive you're asleep is the answer. You have to use your judgment to decide how long you think you sleep for (or use a device such as the Zeo; see box, p.202), but if you think you sleep for only four hours a night, you would reduce your sleep time so that you spend five hours in bed. Lowering overall sleep time in this way in effect artificially manipulates your sleeping patterns. You're awake for longer, so more tired when bedtime comes round. Then, when you do go to bed, your brain quickly finds deep sleep. Periods of deep sleep and dreaming sleep lengthen (to make up the sleep debt of the forced shorter night), so that when you wake in the morning, you feel generally more refreshed than when you spent more time in bed but believed you were sleeping less. Your actual sleep is deeper with fewer awakenings, so there are fewer moments between sleep cycles in which you believe yourself to be awake. Once you've restored your faith in the refreshing powers of your sleep, you can resume more normal sleeping–waking hours.

Fatal familial insomnia

Exactly as its name suggests, fatal familial insomnia (FFI) is an inherited condition (related to a particular gene) that can lead to death. It was the first "sleep disorder" that was found to be associated with a single gene mutation. The gene in question is the prion protein gene (*PRNP*), which is the same gene that can lead to CJD – Creuzfeldt Jakob Disease, the human equivalent of BSE (mad cow disease). Carriers of the abnormal *PRNP* gene are at risk of FFI, but developing the condition is not a certainty.

Studies show that the first sign of this extreme case of insomnia is dramatic weight loss, then a gradual worsening of sleep quality until eventually sleep won't come at all. Damage to the thalamus, the brain's main sensory highway and the area that partly moves into neutral and disengages us from the real world when we fall asleep, means that the sufferer gradually experiences difficulty in falling asleep and then maintaining sleep, ultimately leaving them in a perpetual state of wakefulness. In its latter stages, the disorder causes sufferers to apparently enact dreams (although proper sleep won't come) or become locked in a state of living stupor. Basic brain control systems fail, leading to problems with temperature regulation, sweating and salivation. Eventually, the vital organs start to break down, including the heart and lungs, which leads to death.

There are two forms of the insomnia and both are fatal, taking anything from six months to two years to run their course. In a single case study, one patient was able to undergo anaesthesia, electro-convulsive therapy and light therapy, and remained functional and able to write a book before he died, two years after first showing signs of the disease. Agomelatine, an antidepressant, which has a similar structure to melatonin, may normalize sleep for a time.

Another, similar form of this insomnia is called Sporadic Fatal Insomnia and occurs when the prion protein gene mutates without any inheritance coming into play. In other words, scientists have found incidents in which people have died of fatal insomnia but have shown no inherited predisposition. In these cases the insomnia is caused by infection or arises simply for unknown reasons.

I want to stress that all kinds of fatal insomnia are extremely rare.

NARCOLEPSY

A form of hypersomnia (excessive sleepiness; see box, p.156), narcolepsy is characterized by sudden sleep onset. It occurs relatively rarely, affecting anywhere between 25 and 50 people per 100,000 depending upon which country you're living in. Incidence is very low among Israeli Jews, for example, but higher among the Japanese. The reasons for this are not clear.

Sufferers may or may not feel warning signs that sleep is about to overcome them, but anyway warning makes little difference – falling asleep is impossible to prevent. There are two main types of narcolepsy: with cataplexy (sudden muscle weakness; see box, p.157) and without. Other symptoms may include terrifying hypnagogic hallucinations (see p.181), sleep paralysis (see p.182), automatic behaviour (when you do something and know you must have done it, but have no recollection of doing it) and disrupted nighttime sleep.

Most people first notice symptoms of the condition between the ages of 15 and 25 years old; although a second, smaller peak in cases occurs in people between the ages of 35 and 45, and near menopause in women. The first symptoms are excessive daytime sleepiness and irresistible sleep attacks, both of which might be exacerbated by high room temperatures and boredom.

Causes

Narcolepsy can occur in those with a genetic predisposition to the condition, but your genes don't necessarily mean that you'll definitely become narcoleptic – in fact the condition shows in only two and five percent of those with a family history. Rather we think that in most cases viral assault causes an auto-immune response that in itself destroys wakefulness-promoting neurons in the brain's hypothalamus, which makes it much harder to stay awake. The virus breaks down the cells that manufacture hypocretin or orexin (the same thing with two different names), a form of small protein that allows your neurons to communicate with one another to regulate your sleep–wake cycle. Once these cells are destroyed you become deficient in hypocretin and so susceptible to the sudden, uncontrollable need to sleep.

Narcolepsy is not only genetic, nor is it only an auto-immune condition. We know, for example, that a small group of narcoleptics retain normal levels of hyopcretin and we're still trying to get to the bottom of how their condition comes about.

Diagnosis

If you think you may have narcolepsy, read about the Epworth Sleepiness Scale on page 10. If you try the test and score higher than fifteen, it's very likely that you're experiencing excessive amounts of daytime sleepiness, to the levels we might expect in a narcoleptic.

In order for a doctor to make a diagnosis, he or she will look at your history of daytime sleepiness and may ask you to undergo daytime nap testing at a sleep centre. Taking on average fewer than eight minutes to fall asleep for a nap (indicating low "sleep latency") and having two or more naps that begin with dreaming sleep confirms your diagnosis. The immediate entry into dreaming sleep helps to explain narcolepsy's characteristic hypnagogic hallucinations. You may also need to give a spinal fluid sample from which doctors can measure your hypocretin levels: low levels indicate a high probability of narcolepsy.

SLEEP SCIENCE

OTHER HYPERSOMNIAS

Narcolepsy is just one kind of hypersomnia, but there are several others. They are:

- *Idiopathic hypersomnia*: This is excessive daytime sleepiness without an obvious cause. It is characterized by naps that don't relieve sleepiness, increased "fogginess" when waking from sleep, and increased sleep time to up to 18 hours a day (or any combination of these factors). It usually develops slowly during adolescence, but affects only around fifty people in every million.
- *Recurrent hypersomnia*: This hypersomnia is characterized by excessive daytime sleepiness that may last for several weeks, and then go away. Over the course of a year, a sufferer may have several episodes, but at other times function perfectly normally.
- *Kleine-Levin syndrome*: This extremely rare syndrome causes 18-hour or more sleep episodes for long periods of time. These then resolve themselves and sleeping returns to normal, only to perhaps recur at a later date.
- *Menstrual-related hypersomnia*: This hypersomnia occurs in women, coinciding only with the time of the menstrual period.
- *Behaviourally induced insufficient sleep syndrome*: This is not a biologically related condition, but instead occurs when a person doesn't allow themselves enough time for sleep. People who regularly work double shifts might fall into this category.

Treatments

At the present time, most treatments for narcolepsy are pharmacological. A sleep specialist may prescribe stimulants to overcome daytime sleepiness, and other drugs to manage symptoms of cataplexy, if relevant. In some countries doctors prescribe amphetamines (as narcoleptics will need to take these for life, addiction concerns

SLEEP SCIENCE

CATAPLEXY

Occuring in around two thirds of narcoleptics, cataplexy is defined as muscle weakness that is triggered by laughter, joking, fear, embarrassment or anger. The emotional triggers are remarkably specific – anxiety, for example, is not a trigger; nor is sadness. When an attack occurs, you may feel anything from an inability to smile or move the muscles in your face, to overwhelming weakness in the knees that causes you to fall to the floor, remaining awake and alert the whole time. Attacks usually last for a few minutes – sometimes more – and are often misdiagnosed as epilepsy.

don't apply).

Although it's almost inevitable that you'll need conventional medical intervention to cope with the condition, it may be possible to help manage it at home. Try to make sure you stick to a firm routine of getting up and going to bed. Avoid caffeine (despite its stimulant effects, it gives you a short-term high and then a debilitating crash) and eating big meals and drinking alcohol, which will make you feel sleepy (see pp.35 and 66–7). Keep your room temperature on the cool side (wear an extra sweater if you feel chilly), and if you sense boredom creeping in, get up and take a short walk, or switch to doing something else for a while. Light exercise and fresh air will help to keep sleepiness at bay.

Take regular naps if you can throughout the day, each lasting no more than 30 minutes. Talk to your employer and ask for flexible working or other ways in which you can optimize your working life while accommodating the inevitable limitations of your condition. Good employers will be sympathetic to your needs if you explain – do bear in mind, though, that there's little published information about narcolepsy and you may need to explain a lot. You'll need to tell your country's driving agency about your condition, too. Support groups, such as Narcolepsy UK and Narcolepsy Network in the USA, will offer advice on how best to approach your boss and the authorities.

PARASOMNIAS

A parasomnia is quite simply an unwanted or unexpected behaviour that occurs during sleep. Almost all parasomnias tend to occur during deep or dreaming sleep. Parasomnias happen because sleep is not a single, unified state. During sleep some parts of the brain – particularly the rational parts – can be asleep, while those that control movement and the senses associated with movement can remain active. It's similar to the experience of realizing you've driven a great distance on a quiet stretch of highway without any conscious recollection of what's been happening on the road around you.

Almost all sleep disorders that are not classed as clinical insomnia, a sleep-related breathing disorder or circadian rhythm disorder, nightmares or narcolepsy can be said to be deep-sleep parasomnias. This class of sleep disorder includes:
• Confusional arousals
• Night terrors
• Sleepwalking
• REM behaviour disorder
• Bruxism (teeth-grinding)

They also include the more unusual sleep disorders, such as exploding head syndrome, sexsomnia and sleep-related groaning.

Although parasomnias may be frightening (in the case of terrors or sleep paralysis, in particular), they're not inherently bad for your health. Bruxism may require you to see a dentist, but otherwise the problems are more to do with disturbed sleeping patterns – both of the parasomniac and of those sharing a sleeping space with him or her – and the resulting problems that such disruption might cause for alertness, focus and good mood the following day. It's thought that around ten percent of Americans are affected by parasomnias. Most of them are children, who are more susceptible because of the amount of processing, learning and rewiring going on in the young brain.

The deep-sleep parasomnias themselves have no or relatively sparse mental content. Awakening someone from a parasomnia event will be difficult and slow.

Most parasomnias occur following a period of sleep deprivation – overtired children and adults will immediately dive into deep sleep, for longer than normal periods of time, in order to make up the sleep debt. Other triggers are stress and fever, and, in the case of adults, having drunk alcohol too close to bedtime. Many psychoactive medicines (medicines that cross the blood-brain barrier and act upon the central nervous system), most notably sleeping pills, can provoke parasomniac episodes, particularly episodes of sleepwalking.

Confusional arousals

These occur when you wake up or are woken from sleep feeling disoriented and anxious, often sitting up and possibly talking, shouting, crying or thrashing about, but making no sense. Within a few moments, although it may take as long as half an hour, the arousal passes and you lie back down again as if nothing has happened. In the morning, you don't tend to remember the episode, although you might remember a brief moment of waking if you're reminded of it.

Confusional arousals are especially common in childhood. They're mainly hereditary – children of a parent who had these arousals frequently as a child are up to 40 percent more susceptible. This rises to 60 percent if both parents were sufferers. When confusional arousals occur in adults, they're often associated with violent behaviour.

Gentle, soothing reassurances should help settle the sleeper back down without incident, and there's certainly no benefit that we yet know of for waking him or her up.

Night terrors

Also occurring most often during childhood, and also mainly inherited, night terrors are sudden, terrified arousals from deep sleep that you then don't remember in the morning. They usually occur during the first three to four hours of sleep and are distinct from nightmares, which occur during lighter, dreaming sleep and which the dreamer

SLEEP CLINIC

My wife says that I groan as I sleep. Am I just snoring or am I having a nightmare?

Snoring is a distinct sound, and if your wife is saying that you're groaning, it's possible that you have a rare parasomnia called sleep-related groaning, or catathrenia. Sounds range from groans, to moans, hums, cracks, squeaks and even roars. The disorder mostly occurs in men, usually beginning in childhood or adolescence.

One way to be more sure of your diagnosis is to work out when the sounds begin and how long they go on for. Sleep-related groaning usually starts at about two hours into sleep (as we enter the first period of dreaming sleep) and each sound may last anything from a few seconds to a minute, as the sleeper is breathing out. Sounds tend to cluster, and each cluster may last up to an hour.

As for whether or not you're having a nightmare, only you can really say – but sufferers of sleep-related groaning rarely have anguished expressions on their faces as they make their sounds, so I think it's unlikely. Tell your wife that if she nudges you in the ribs to force you to change your sleeping position, you're likely to stop.

usually recalls on waking.

Watching someone go through a night terror can in itself be a frightening experience. The sleeper may thrash, kick, scream and lash out, demonstrating a sense of panic that seems utterly real. He or she probably won't know who you are if you begin talking them.

Make sure the sleeper is safe, but don't try to wake them. Stay close until the episode has passed (it may take anything from a few minutes to half an hour) and, only once you're sure it's over, gently rouse them from their sleep if you can. It's thought that waking the sleeper at this point may help to prevent them going straight back into deep sleep with the possibility of another night terror episode. If the terror occurs at the same time every night, you could try waking the sleeper shortly before this time comes round. In doing so, you hope to break the cycle and this way prevent the night terror happening at all.

Sleepwalking

Although we call it sleepwalking, somnambulation is actually far more than just walking. Any complex, automated or instinctive behaviour that occurs when you're fully asleep – from sitting up in bed, to walking into another room, to picking up the remote control and staring at the TV (with or without turning it on), and even driving a car (it has been known!) – falls under the umbrella term sleepwalking.

Sleepwalkers have no memory of their behaviour and are usually so deeply asleep during each episode that they're hard to rouse, and may even become aggressive or argumentative if you try. Nonetheless, if the sleepwalker is in any danger (if, for example, he or she goes out to get into a car), it's essential to prevent them from pursuing their mission.

Although sleepwalking occurs mostly during childhood (and children will usually grow out of it), it's also one of the more common parasomnias for adults. The good news is that the only dangers it brings are the health and safety issues of what you might do while you're moving and asleep. There are no links that we know of between sleepwalking and other, more sinister mental or psychological disorders.

If you want to encourage a sleepwalker back to bed, I've found that putting a rough, hessian-type doormat at the exit to a bedroom can help. The sensation of the mat beneath bare feet triggers the realization that this is the way out of the bedroom and hopefully results in an about-turn. If you yourself are a sleepwalker, try standing on the mat before you go to bed and saying to yourself, "If I feel this beneath my feet, I must return to bed!" Anecdotally, some people have found that a big sign on the bedroom door that reads, "Go back to bed!" is enough to make the sleepwalker do exactly that. Behavioural approaches, such as both these, are better, in my opinion, than resorting to medication, although short, two-week courses of antidepressants have been shown to reduce sleepwalking episodes among students.

SLEEP SCIENCE

SEXSOMNIA

In recent years, I've been called as an expert witness in a number of sexsomnia cases. This rare parasomnia results in a person engaging in sexual activity during sleep that he or she doesn't then remember. Sexsomnia occurs mostly during deep sleep, although it may also occur during light stages. Both men and women might suffer, and even couples can together discover that they've been having intercourse in their sleep without realizing it. Intercourse isn't the only sexual activity that may occur – sleep masturbation and sleep fondling are also types of sexsomnia.

Owing to the delicate nature of the disorder, it's essential that anyone who thinks they might suffer from sexsomnia takes steps to ensure they don't endanger anyone else. Although sadly it's virtually impossible to know you have the condition until you advance on another person, if you suffer from other parasomnias or have obstructive sleep apnoea, and are overtired or have drunk too much alcohol, you're more likely to have a sexsomniac episode, too. Usual treatments for parasomniacs (see below), as well as clonazepam, a benzodiazepine medication (see p.189), may help.

REM Behaviour Disorder

In normal periods of REM, dreams occur only in the sleeper's imagination. We can do wonderful things in the world of dreams, but we act out none of those things in reality because the communication channels between our brain and our muscles have closed down for the night. For a person suffering from REM Behaviour Disorder (RBD) this natural and necessary breakdown in communication doesn't occur, meaning that sufferers can act out their dreams. In many cases RBD sufferers become violent.

One possible explanation for RBD is that dreaming sleep switches on too early, before the previous sleep stage is fully over and while the brain is still in the process of creating the temporary state of paralysis that characterizes R sleep. Or, it might switch on too late, while the brain is beginning to start up communication with our muscles again. Either of these scenarios would certainly explain how RBD comes about, but we're still a long way from being certain that one or other (or both) is what's going on.

It's thought that about half a percent of the general population suffer from RBD. Initially, scientists believed that it affected mainly older men (around 90 percent of cases occurring in men over the age of fifty), but more recent research has shown that it may also occur in younger women. We don't yet know why, except that RBD is also more common among people who take antidepressant medication – which tends to be women more often than men. Autoimmune disease such as multiple sclerosis or the combination of an autoimmune and inflammatory disease (such as arthritis), as well as narcolepsy and Parkinson's Disease, all seem to have links with RBD – but we're still trying to resolve how these links work and what they mean. The good news is that as a disorder in itself, RBD is relatively easy to treat.

If you think you may suffer from RBD, you'll need to see your doctor and visit a sleep clinic for a firm diagnosis. Only in clinic conditions can we determine that you're suffering from lack of muscle paralysis during periods of R and therefore be certain that you have RBD rather than another parasomnia. Once diagnosed, your doctor will probably offer you psychoactive medication, such as clonazepam, which has muscle relaxant, anticonvulsive and sedative properties. This medication works in 90 percent of cases to eradicate RBD altogether.

For your safety and for the safety of the people you live with, it's essential that you seek help for this condition. In the meantime, remove all sharp objects in the vicinity of your bed, and don't sleep in a loft bed or near a window. Until you've overcome the parasomnia, you must make yourself and those around you safe.

Bruxism

First described in 1907, bruxism is characterized by jaw clenching, and by teeth grinding that may or may not be noisy. It occurs mainly during light sleep and rarely during deep and dreaming sleep. Sufferers may experience an average of 170 episodes a night and in the morning may wake up with a headache and a tense, sore jaw, aching face muscles and even ear ache. Some of these symptoms can become chronic – lasting well beyond the waking hours and worsening over time. Of course, that's not to mention the effects of wear on the teeth and jaw, and the fact that eating breakfast can become somewhat uncomfortable, or even painful. In the long term, bruxism can disrupt the sleep of both the sufferer and anyone with whom he or she shares a room. Three out of four sufferers report that they feel sleepy during the daytime.

Bruxism has interesting physiological effects on the body. At around four to eight minutes prior to an episode, your heart starts to beat more forcibly (as if you were preparing to fight or flee from danger), and then a few seconds before you start to grind your teeth, your brainwaves reach alpha-wave frequency – as if you've risen to wakefulness. However, this burst of alpha activity is too short to be scored as true wakefulness – it's over within seconds, followed by another rise in heart rate and then the grinding and gnashing.

The condition is surprisingly common with an estimated 80 to 85 percent of the population clenching or grinding their teeth at some point in their lives. Studies show that bruxism is often triggered during periods of stress and anxiety, but there are other risk factors for the disorder. If you already have another sleep disorder, including snoring, obstructive sleep apnoea or another parasomnia, you're thought to be at greater risk of developing bruxism, too. Smokers and heavy drinkers are also at risk, as well as those taking certain medications, including haloperidol, lithium, chlorpromazine and methylphenidate. Those who have epilepsy, Huntingdon's disease, Parkinson's disease and Tourette's syndrome are also at risk.

Without a cure for bruxism, we need instead to look at ways to manage the disorder. There's modest evidence that behavioural approaches can help. These include understanding the causes and the factors that exacerbate the condition and taking steps to reverse the habit of clenching and grinding the teeth. For example, some people find controlled abdominal breathing can help (see box, opposite).

SLEEP THERAPY

ABDOMINAL BREATHING FOR BRUXISM

Overcoming the habit of clenching your teeth is a good first step to reducing your likelihood of a bruxism attack. In this exercise, the in- and outbreath and the rise and fall of your abdomen are linked with letting go tension in your jaw. Practise it every day before you go to bed. You'll need a paperback book.

1. Lie comfortably on your back on the floor on a large towel or a yoga mat if you have one. Place the book on your chest, then gently rest your hands, palms down by your sides on the floor.

2. Close your eyes and become conscious of how you're holding your jaw – is it tight? Are your teeth clenched? Is your tongue rigid or loose inside your mouth? Try to release any tension in your mouth and jaw – you may notice a tingling sensation in your cheeks and temples as you let go.

3. Now turn your attention to your breath. Breathe in through your nose as far as you can. As you breathe in, become conscious of the book rising on your chest, then as the breath reaches your abdomen push upward, letting your abdomen rise slightly higher than the book on your chest. This fully expands your diaphragm. Hold for one second.

4. Breathe out through your mouth and notice how your abdomen and then the book lower. As you exhale, allow your lower jaw to fall open, consciously releasing any tension there.

5. Continue breathing in and out like this for ten minutes. Take care not to overbreathe (if you become dizzy, stop and breathe normally for a bit). After five to ten breaths you should feel the tension release from your whole face, as well as from your jaw.

Improved sleep hygiene and any therapy that helps to relieve stress are also positive ways to help overcome bruxism.

In conventional treatment, a dentist can fit a mouthguard, a mandibular advancement device (see pp.177–8) or a bite splint to protect your teeth. In time we may also be able to prescribe devices that send an electrical vibration into the mouth to prevent grinding; solutions, however, are currently only at trial stage. Stress-relief medications and medications to regulate serotonin levels may also help.

General prevention and treatment for parasomnias

No matter what parasomnia you may suffer from, you'll be unaware of what you're doing and usually have no (or perhaps only patchy) memory of what has happened. If it's your child who's suffering, given that the episodes rarely cause any long-term stress or health issues, I recommend that you do nothing about them at all. By the time your child has reached young adulthood, it's very likely that he or she won't experience parasomniac episodes any more.

In adults the situation is more complex. While there appears to be no underlying health issue for most parasomniac activity, parasomniacs are potentially a danger to themselves and other household members. At the very least, they'll disturb the sleep of those around them.

It may be possible to reduce the number of episodes in both adults and children by having good sleep hygiene. Take special care to:

- Create a well-defined and calming bedtime routine, so that bedtime is a happy, quiet and reassuring experience. (This goes for adults as well as children.)
- Make sure you spend some time relaxing and unwinding before you go to bed (stress might cause an episode).
- Avoid situations that might result in over-tiredness or sleep deprivation. This means having a sleep–wake schedule that you stick to every day of the week.

CIRCADIAN RHYTHM SLEEP DISORDERS

As we've already seen, the time at which each of us falls asleep is dictated by two main things. First, how tired we are, which comes as a result of our activity levels during the day, how long we've been awake previously and the efficiency of the previous night's sleep and, second, the ticking of the biological clock.

Your biological clock runs slightly more slowly than real-time hours during the day, and speeds up slightly at dawn. The overall result is that the body is generally in sync with the 24-hour calendar day. If, however, the clock runs too quickly or too slowly, your body steps out of real time, and your sleep may not begin or end when it "should" – that is, the time that society or your lifestyle requires you to be asleep. It's important to note that, once asleep, those with only a circadian rhythm sleep disorder and no other sleep disorder will experience normal sleeping patterns. In other words, it's the sleeping and waking times that become a problem, rather than the sleep quality itself.

Circadian rhythm sleep disorders are also known as biological clock disorders and subcategorized as the following types:

- *Phase delay*, or delayed sleep phase type: the clock runs slowly and out of kilter, on a repeating pattern (a "fixed delay"), creating an extreme "owl" (see box, p.17).
- *Phase advance*, or advanced sleep phase type: the clock runs quickly and out of kilter, creating an extreme "lark".
- *Irregular sleep–wake type*: the clock runs erratically, causing tiredness at inappropriate times, although in all the sufferer gets the "right" amount of sleep in 24 hours.
- *Free-running (non-entrained) type*: the clock always runs slowly (continuously delaying), so that the sufferer has no regular falling asleep time, nor wake-up time, as the biological clock delays the onset of sleepiness by a little more every day. It can take a couple of weeks for a sufferer to come back to a "normal" sleep time, and for the cycle of delay to start again.
- *Jet-lag type*: the clock runs at a different time to the local time zone (see pp.112–6).
- *Shift-work type*: the clock runs at a different time to the sleep–

wake schedule as dictated by shift rotas (see pp.105–8).

Causes

Delayed, advanced, irregular and free-running disorders in adults can occur as a result of injury, stroke, disease, or even genetic abnormalities that manifest only with age. Problems with receptor cells in the retina, the optic nerve, melatonin secretion, any of the pathways that transmit light information to the biological clock, as well as problems with the biological clock itself, are all possible causes.

In adolescents, the onset of phase delay is to do with growing up – a by-product of puberty (it may last for several years after puberty itself is over). The biological clock slows down, delaying the secretion of melatonin to trigger sleep. See pages 81–5 for more information specifically related to the sleep of adolescents.

Treatments

Unless it's obvious which type of circadian rhythm sleep disorder you have (as it would be for jet lag or shift work), the best way to diagnose your problem is to keep a sleep diary for two to four weeks. Carefully recording your sleeping, waking and napping (if relevant) times, as well as the levels of daytime tiredness you feel, will help you to see whether or not you're running slower or faster than the 24-hour clock. Once you have a better idea how your body clock is working, you can set about trying to reset your sleep–wake rhythm.

Making changes to a physiological problem with the biological clock, whatever its cause, is not straightforward, but the key is the use of light. This is because the biggest cue for the biological clock is changing light. Other cues, such as exercise and mealtimes, may help, but are less fundamental to how the internal clock keeps time.

An old-fashioned approach to resolving phase delay was to force the sleeper to push forward their sleep onset time by two to three hours a night until they arrived again at the "right" time for going to sleep – usually between 10pm and midnight. For example, if you don't usually feel sleepy until around 2am, you'd spend several nights moving that sleep onset time on by two to three hours (so, 2am one night, then 4am the following night and so on, each time sleeping for the "right" number of hours), until you reached, say, a sleep time of 10pm. At this point you'd have reset your clock so that you fell asleep at the appropriate time. The problem with this approach on its own is that phase delay keeps going, and the desire to fall asleep late just starts all over again.

If, though, you can combine the approach with the use of bright light, you may be able to keep the new schedule relatively under control. So, choosing a period when you can dedicate several days to the sleep-onset process, reset your clock so that you fall asleep at an appropriate time. Then in the morning get good exposure to bright light (ideally sunlight) to help your body to embed the new schedule. As with coping with jet lag (see pp.112–6), getting up and out for a morning run or a brisk walk is a good start. You could also buy a light box – many light boxes are available that have been specifically designed to overcome this type of sleep disorder.

The system works the opposite way round for phase advance. Bring forward your bedtime by two to three hours every night until you have worked back to the appropriate time for going to sleep. To avoid slipping out of kilter again, expose yourself to bright light in the evening. This can be as simple as taking an early evening walk (or mid-afternoon in winter) or run (not fewer than four hours before bedtime), or flooding your home with light, even if it's artificial. Again, a specially dedicated light box is ideal.

Free-running and irregular sleep–wake types simply have to adapt the principles for phase advance and delay so that they, too, begin to follow a clear bedtime and waking time. Do all you can to avoid napping, so that you're tired at "normal" bedtime, and use light exposure to help.

In all cases, it can take several months for the biological clock to find its new, improved rhythm, so it's essential that you're prepared to stick rigidly for a long time to the schedule changes you put in place. Avoid using alcohol as a means to help you to fall asleep (see pp.66–7), and it may help to go caffeine-free (and avoid any other stimulants for that matter), certainly while you're trying to reset your clock. Also bear in mind that some medications include stimulants and you may not realize that these are disrupting your ability to fall asleep. Talk to your doctor if this may be the case for you.

Finally, your doctor may advise that you take a melatonin supplement. There's great debate about how this works and how effective it is, although on paper the signs are certainly good: the supplement resets the biological clock and may promote sleep at the appropriate time. I recommend giving this a go under professional supervision if the more natural, schedule-related efforts don't work. (See box, p.116.)

SLEEP-RELATED BREATHING DISORDERS

Although you might think that you breathe more deeply and peacefully while you sleep, generally the opposite is true. When you're in non-dreaming sleep, your breathing does become more regular, but it's also more shallow. An exciting dream may upset this pattern, causing sharper, more raspy and irregular breaths.

All this is perfectly normal, and shouldn't disrupt your sleep or be any cause for concern. However, if, during sleep, your breathing is laboured or noisy (snoring), or if it's very shallow (hypopnoea), or if you have short periods in which your breathing stops altogether (apnoea), and in any of these situations you wake up feeling unrefreshed, you may have a sleep-related breathing disorder.

Snoring

Many couples I meet resort to sleeping in different rooms when one of them is a regular snorer. Unfortunately, snoring is often as disturbing for the listener as it is for the sufferer, but that's not the only reason to do something about it. The grunting sound can indicate several underlying conditions that it's important you check out.

Snoring is the result of a vibration of the tissues of your airways as you sleep. This vibration occurs because you have some sort of respiratory obstruction – which might be anything from the build-up of fatty tissue around your throat to the result of sleeping on your back, which causes your tongue to drop backward and partially block your airways. Phlegm or mucus can also cause obstruction, which is why you might tend to snore if you have a cold.

Temporary (acute) snoring, with a distinct cause, such as tonsillitis or cold, is not necessarily a problem and will pass once the illness abates or has been treated. If you snore because of your sleeping position, usually an elbow in the ribs from your partner will soon put that to rights. However, if snoring is chronic – that is, it's prolonged and sustained – you need to do something about it. Up to 40 percent of chronic snorers have significantly disturbed sleep that negatively affects their mood, ability to focus, and libido. Statistics also show that snorers have a ten-fold increase in the risk of a stroke. Furthermore, specialists in respiration believe that snoring may mask a more serious condition, such as obstructive sleep apnoea.

Obstructive sleep apnoea

When a total blockage of the airways causes your breathing to stop for ten seconds or more, you have obstructive sleep apnoea (OSA). OSA is probably the most prevalent sleep disorder of the twentieth century – but it has been known for hundreds of years. Today, we estimate that around four in every hundred middle-aged men and two in every hundred middle-aged women suffer from OSA.

All manner of problems can cause the blockage, including ana-tomical factors such as collapse of your throat or pharynx owing to excessive fat around your neck, enlarged tonsils or adenoids, the base of your tongue being larger than normal, or having poorly aligned jaws. Smoking causes inflammation, swelling and narrowing of the airways in the throat, and various medical disorders can make the problem worse, including nasal congestion, hypothyroidism, acromegaly (too much growth hormone), vocal cord paralysis, Marfan's syndrome (an inherited disorder of the connective tissue), Down's syndrome and neuromuscular disorders.

What happens during OSA

During sleep, sometimes more than once every minute, the blockage obstructs your airways causing cessation in breathing. As soon as your body detects that it's being starved of oxygen, you're brought instantly into a lighter stage of sleep, or sometimes a very brief period of wakefulness, in order to restore normal breathing – if only temporarily. That little awakening is called an "arousal" – it's not enough to wake you fully, but it's enough to disturb your sleep. Clinicians grade OSA according to the number of times a night you experience an arousal:

• Five to 14 interruptions per hour: mild OSA.
• 15 to 30 interruptions per hour: moderate OSA.
• More than 30 interruptions per hour: severe OSA.

The unit of measurement for these breathing impairments is the "apnoea–hypoponea index", and systems for measuring where you fall on the index vary from country to country. The gold standard for measurement is to use a polysomnography – a system available at sleep centres that records your brainwaves, eye movements and muscle tone during sleep. In addition, technicians can measure nasal air-flow, snoring, and blood-oxygen levels. If you have suspected severe OSA, you may be given a sensor kit to use at home, which measures nasal air-flow and blood-oxygen levels, or chest straps to measure your breathing rate.

In some people OSA interruptions are so frequent that sufferers experience no deep sleep at all. The result is further fatigue, leading to reduced daytime performance, a general inability to concentrate, and excessive daytime sleepiness (given the term OSA Syndrome). In these cases activities such as driving are extremely dangerous. There are also physiological effects of OSA. Regular, intermittent breaks in oxygen to the brain can have lasting effects on the brain's make-up, leading to a stroke. Breathing impairment is associated with major changes in blood pressure, and the entire scenario may ultimately lead to long-term damage in your heart, brain, and blood vessels.

The good news is that, once diagnosed, OSA is perfectly treatable. (Be aware that if you're diagnosed with OSA, you'll need to let your insurance company know, as well as your driving licence issuer.)

SLEEP SCIENCE

OSA: SIGNS AND SYMPTOMS

- Daytime fatigue and/or sleepiness
- Loud snoring
- Morning headaches
- A dry mouth on waking
- Irritability
- Changes in personality
- Depression
- Difficulty in concentrating
- Frequent visits to the loo at night
- Excessive perspiration during sleep
- Heartburn
- Reduced libido

Other types of sleep apnoea

OSA is not the only form of sleep apnoea. The following are less common, but worth mentioning and certainly worth investigating if you think one of them is affecting you.

Central sleep apnoea occurs when the brain fails to send appropriate signals to the breathing muscles to maintain respiration during sleep. It's often associated with a central nervous system disease that involves a blockage or infection in the lower parts of the brain. It can also occur in neuromuscular diseases that involve the respiratory muscles – I've seen it most in patients with multiple sclerosis.

Mixed sleep apnoea results from a mix of both central sleep apnoea and OSA. Usually the central sleep apnoea (which is not caused by any obstruction) is quickly followed by an airway obstruction. This is more common than central sleep apnoea, but less common than OSA.

Upper airway resistance syndrome (UARS) is a term that was coined by US sleep researcher and physician Christian Guilleminault in 1993. UARS is characterized by repetitive arousals from sleep that probably

OSA: WHO'S MOST AT RISK?

Evidence suggests that OSA is worse if you are elderly, male or overweight. As we age, throat muscle slowly turns to fat, which may begin to obstruct the airways. The reasons why in general men have a higher risk of OSA than women is not entirely clear. Post-menopausal women (who have proportionately lower levels of the female hormone oestrogen than women who are pre-menopause) are at a higher risk of OSA than younger women.

Weight has a significant influence on susceptibility to OSA. If you've already developed mild forms of the condition, be aware that only a one-percent increase in body weight leads to a three-percent increase in the risk that you'll develop moderate or severe OSA. With a ten-percent increase in body weight, the risk is six-fold. If you're obese or have a collar size of greater than 40cm (16in), you're particularly susceptible to OSA.

result from increasing respiratory effort during narrowing of the upper airway. While this may result in snoring, the condition is distinct from OSA and hypopnoea in that it doesn't affect the levels of oxygen present in the blood. Because there's no actual break in breathing, oxygen levels are maintained. Nevertheless, UARS patients suffer the same levels of effective sleep disruption as other apnoea patients. There is, though, much controversy among experts as to whether UARS is a specific syndrome or part of a spectrum of obstructive disorders affecting the upper airway.

Treatments for sleep-related breathing disorders

If you suffer from any form of sleep-related breathing disorder, you should avoid alcohol and sleeping pills. These drugs dull your brain's arousal mechanism, making it harder for you to have the little awakenings that are essential for your intake of oxygen. Alcohol also relaxes the muscles that may be obstructing your airways, sometimes making even mild conditions, such as snoring, considerably worse.

Optimize your sleep hygiene so that you have every chance of a good night's sleep, despite your sleep disorder. Studies show that there are fewer incidences of OSA when sufferers are well rested.

If you're overweight it's essential that you lose weight, as this will almost certainly improve your chances of overcoming all kinds of sleep-related breathing disorder. Try some throat exercises, too, to tighten up the muscles in the back of your throat, helping to prevent collapse. See the box on page 176 for some exercises to try.

Thereafter, there are several medical devices (listed below) that your clinician may suggest for you, or you may require surgery.

Nasal airstrips

If you're a snorer because you have restricted airflow through your nasal passages, you might find that nasal airstrips (available in most pharmacies) provide a simple and non-invasive solution to your problem. You attach the strips over the bridge of your nose, which has the effect of opening your nostrils and airways so that you can breathe through your nose more easily. Nasal dilators and saline sprays can also help by having the same effects.

Continuous Positive Airway Pressure (CPAP)

A CPAP is a nose and mouth mask that is connected to an air blower. A common form of treatment for all breathing disorders, from snoring to OSA, it forces air into your lungs raising the air pressure (usually automatically) in your mouth, nose and throat just enough to prevent your airways from collapsing. Although initial CPAP devices (brought out in the early 1980s) were big and heavy, modern systems are often small enough even to be taken on aircraft. You may also hear it called an nCPAP (nasal CPAP, which covers just the nose) or a BiPAP (BiLevel Positive Airway Pressure), which adjusts the air pressure both for inspiration and for expiration.

The pitfalls of CPAP include:

SLEEP THERAPY

STRENGTHENING YOUR MOUTH AND THROAT

A study in the USA in 2009 revealed that a group of snorers and OSA sufferers asked to do 30 minutes of throat exercises every day for three months reduced their symptoms by almost 40 percent. Practise the following once a day (you don't have to do them all in the same session) and see if your symptoms improve over time.

1. Using your toothbrush, scrub away at the centre and sides of your tongue for three minutes a day. This action triggers the gagging reflex, which has the effect of tensing and releasing your throat muscles and tongue to help strengthen them.
2. Suck in your cheeks as hard as you can. Hold and release, then repeat. Do this for three minutes.
3. Put your index finger against the inside of one cheek and suck in the other cheek hard. Practise for three minutes on each side.
4. Lick the roof of your mouth with the tip of your tongue from front to back (as far as you can go). Do this for three minutes.
5. Open your mouth wide and let out a series of short "ah" sounds, followed by one continuous "ahhh". Repeat for three minutes.
6. Place a deflated balloon to your lips, then breathe in through your nose and out through your mouth, aiming to inflate the balloon as much as possible with your out-breath. Repeat for three to five times, taking care not to overbreathe.
7. Chew your food on one side of your mouth and then the other. When you swallow, keep your teeth together and jaw closed.

- Nasal congestion and a sore or dry mouth
- Chest muscle discomfort, but this goes away eventually
- Eye irritation
- Irritation and sores over the bridge of the nose
- Nosebleeds

• Upper respiratory infections
• A feeling of being closed in (claustrophobia)

However, the benefits far outweigh the pitfalls. Regular use of CPAP lowers raised blood pressure; improves concentration, alertness, productivity, mood and libido; restores normal sleeping patterns; and reduces anxiety. Your partner may get a better night's sleep, too.

Once your sleep physician has prescribed a CPAP, he or she will select the particular device that most suits your condition; a suitably qualified technician or nurse will choose your mask. I often think the most important aspect of successful therapy is the mask fitting and education session. With the right mask, correctly fitted, you're likely to have a comfortable night that means you wake in the morning feeling bright and alert.

Oral appliances

The term "oral appliance" (also used in dentistry) is given to any device placed in your mouth to modify the position of your jaw, tongue and other structures in the upper airways to reduce snoring and/or sleep apnoea. In the USA, the American Food and Drug Administration has endorsed more than 34 appliances for use in the treatment of OSA.

There are two oral appliances that are most commonly prescribed. It's essential that if you're to have one or other of them, the appliance is moulded, aligned and fitted properly for your mouth. This usually means that a specialist will take a silicone mould that gives accurate measurements of your bite and jaw alignment.

Tongue-retaining devices are useful for patients who have very large tongues, no teeth, poor dental health, suffer from chronic joint pain, or find their sleep apnoea is worse when they're lying on their backs. They aren't suitable for people who are more than 50 percent above their ideal body weight, grind their teeth at night, or have chronically stuffy noses. The tongue retaining device is essentially a mouthguard with a polyvinyl "bubble" sticking out between the upper and lower teeth mould. You hold the device in place by slotting your teeth into the upper and lower mouthguard sections and then you place your tongue into the bubble. As you push in your tongue, a natural vacuum secures it in a forward position so that it can no longer fall back and cause a blockage.

Mandibular advancement devices combine a mouthguard and a dental brace, and attach to your teeth to position your jaw forward slightly as you sleep. The aim is to modify the anatomy of your upper airway, in order to enlarge it, or stabilize or reduce its collapsibility. In this way a mandibular advancement device may reduce snoring and relieve mild sleep apnoea. Some people find that their jaw aches after the first few nights of wearing the device, but usually any discomfort passes as you get more used to it.

Surgery

Snoring and milder forms of OSA may be caused by anatomical deformities that have been present since you were born or are the result of injury to your throat. For some this means that the most effective treatment is surgery. The procedure is most likely to be uvulopalatopharyngoplasty – something of a mouthful in itself! It's a laser surgery that removes excess tissue at the back of the throat and in this way clears the airways. It can take a few weeks or more to get over the sore throat that results from the surgery, but the procedure is effective for up to 75 percent of snoring cases. (More extensive surgery may remove the tonsils, adenoids, or tissue flaps, too.) If you aren't keen on the idea, you may opt for a CPAP (see pp.175–7) instead.

A newer form of surgery is called the Pillar Procedure, which can be performed under local anaesthetic in only 20 minutes. Patients have three small staple-like implants put into the soft palate at the top of the back of the mouth. These implants reduce the vibrations that cause snoring and may help to reduce the level of collapse in the airways to relieve cases of mild OSA. If the procedure doesn't work (not everyone's anatomy is suited to it), surgeons can remove the implants.

RESTLESS LEG SYNDROME

In the mid-20th century, the Swedish neurologist Karl Ekbom clinically identified a condition that had been described in literature for centuries. He called it Ekbom's Syndrome – the sensation of creepy crawlies scuttling over and inside the legs. The condition affects around ten percent of the general population. Some people say the sensations are painful, jittery and tingly. Almost all say that walking around is the only way to relieve them. In sleep clinics we call this Restless Leg Syndrome (RLS), the most common movement-related sleep disorder.

The sensations usually begin late in the evening or at any time until around midnight or just after. They aren't felt just on the skin, but deep within the thigh and calf muscle, and around 50 percent of sufferers feel them in their arms and through other areas of their body, too. Relief comes through movement and may last for up to 30 minutes before the sensations start again, eventually dissipating over a number of hours, often just as the early hours of the morning creep in.

Causes

We still don't really know why RLS should occur when it does. It may be that we move around less toward the end of the day, so the leg muscles suddenly feel that they need to expend some energy. Some evidence suggests that RLS is caused by melatonin secretion (as darkness falls) itself.

The syndrome is partly inherited, with immediate relatives of sufferers being between three and five times more likely to develop it. However, it can also occur by itself, or appear in people who have kidney problems, peripheral nerve damage, coeliac disease or Crohn's disease. Pregnant women often complain of it, although we think that it's pregnancy that may reveal the condition or that RLS reflects poorer absorption of iron from the gut. In children, there appears to be a link with Attention Deficit Hyperactivity Disorder (ADHD).

Finally, we also know that there's a link between RLS and low levels of iron in the bloodstream. These levels don't have to be abnormally low (you don't have to be so deficient in iron as to be anaemic), just low, which means anything below 45 μ/L of iron in your blood. (Ask

SLEEP CLINIC

I get RLS before I go to bed at night, but during the night I'm told that I also jiggle my ankles. Are the two related?

Very possibly. The majority of people who have RLS also have a condition known as periodic limb movements during sleep (PLMS), or nocturnal myoclonus. Usually the limb movements begin with an extension of the muscles of the big toe, which then becomes a flexing of the ankle. Some people even begin flexing their knee and hip. The movements of PLMS are usually not enough for you to become conscious of them, but they are enough to disturb your sleep and probably make you feel quite sleepy the following day. This is why it's important to take steps to deal with the RLS, and so resolve the PLMS and restore better sleep.

your doctor for a blood test to assess your levels of ferritin – the iron transporter.) Iron is also essential for the metabolism of dopamine, a neurotransmitter, low levels of which may also be indicated in RLS.

Treatments

If you suffer from RLS, avoid alcohol and caffeine and generally make sure that you have good sleep hygiene (see Chapter 3). In particular, being overtired can exacerbate the symptoms. If your levels of iron are low, take a daily iron supplement, along with a dose of vitamin C to help iron absorption. However, note that it may take several months of supplementation for RLS symptoms to abate, because it takes this long for the brain to reorganize its iron stores.

If your symptoms persist and are frequent (which means that they occur every day), your doctor may prescribe you with medications such as dopaminergic agents, benzodiazepines (see p.189–90) or opiods to help ease the symptoms.

ISOLATED SYMPTOMS, NORMAL VARIANTS AND UNRESOLVED ISSUES

This rather unwieldy name for a category of sleep disorders actually quite neatly sums up the miscellany that falls under it. Sleeptalking is one of the most common sleep disorders in this category, and affects most of us at some time or another, but isolated symptoms *et al* also includes other common issues such as sleep starts (the jerky movements we sometimes get as we fall asleep) and the rather more scary problem of sleep paralysis.

Sleep starts, terrifying hypnagogic hallucinations and false awakenings

Also known as hypnic or hypnagogic jerks, *sleep starts* are sudden spasms of the legs, arms, face or neck that occur as you fall asleep. Most people experience them at least once in a lifetime – often more. The spasms can be associated with a brief but vivid dream or with the illusion of suddenly falling. Other sensory flashes can occur, as well as complex hallucinations. None of these experiences is harmful and they are not an indication of anything sinister.

A much rarer form of sleep start is the "sensory sleep start", or exploding head syndrome. In this, you experience an apparently very loud, sudden but imagined noise, rather like a violent explosion in your head, sometimes accompanied by leg jerks. Again, the experience is perfectly benign and we think that it's associated with a window of wakefulness, immediately before we fall asleep.

Terrifying hypnagogic hallucinations can occur on their own or during a sleep start. They are distinct from nightmares because they occur in the semi-conscious state that you have as you fall asleep – in the space, as it were, between waking and sleeping. Rather like terrifying dreams, though, the hallucinations often feature attack and aggression, exacerbated by your inability to call for help. Commonly, you lose sense of time, thinking the hallucination has lasted far longer than it actually has. There are some links between terrifying hypnagogic hallucinations and narcolepsy (see pp.154–7), so if you have a lot of these sleep experiences, it may be worth consulting your doctor to see if you're susceptible to narcolepsy, too.

Finally, many people from time to time have a *false awakening*. This rather confusing phenomenon occurs in two forms. In the first, and more common, dream imagery indicates that you've woken up, got dressed, and so on. When something happens that is out of kilter with reality, you're alerted to the fact that you're dreaming and you jolt awake. The second, more alarming type is linked with feelings of foreboding, stress and fear. People who have this kind of false awakening may report seeing monsters, apparitions or strangers. In extreme cases these awakenings are associated with out-of-body experiences.

Neither type of false awakening has any health implications and neither is any cause for real concern. Checking up on your sleep hygiene should help minimize how often they happen to you.

Sleep paralysis

If REM Behaviour Disorder (see pp.161–3) is the result of a system failure resulting in the muscles not disengaging during sleep, sleep paralysis is the opposite. This frightening sleep disorder, which renders the victim conscious but unable to move or speak, usually occurs in the morning as you come out of dreaming (R) sleep. As we already know, your muscles become paralyzed during R. When sleep paralysis occurs, you've come out of your dream into consciousness before the temporary cessation in communication with your muscles has passed.

Another theory suggests that the paralysis is, in fact, all part of a hallucination – which might help to account for some of the feelings that sufferers claim during sleep paralysis episodes. These include feelings of oppression or pressure on the chest, or being violently beaten or choked.

Each episode lasts only a few minutes and adolescents are the most susceptible, although episodes can occur at any time in our lives. (It's thought that all adults will experience an episode at some time.) Sleep researchers have identified several triggers for sleep paralysis, including being overtired, jet lag, depression, stress, overwork, and lying on one's back. As with so many of the parasomnias, sleep paralysis is likely to run in families. It's completely harmless, except for being frightening. If you're a sufferer, read Chapter 3 on sleep hygiene again and optimize all the conditions for your sleep. In most cases, good sleep hygiene will reduce your likelihood of suffering episodes in the future.

NIGHTMARES

Rozalind Cartwright, of Rush University, Chicago, notes that dreams range on a continuum that begins with pleasant dreams and takes us through neutral dreams, less than pleasant dreams, bad dreams and nightmares – the worst kind of dreams. Usually occurring in the second half of the night, nightmares force you awake, often in some state of distress – although very quickly you'll understand what's happened and regain your connection with reality. Nonetheless, you may find it hard to go back to sleep, haunted by your frightening visions.

A nightmare usually involves a sense of fear, anxiety or panic; a threat to survival, security or self-esteem and dysphoric emotions such as anger, sadness or disgust. Although we may think of nightmares as a disorder of very young children, in fact their prevalence increases between pre-school age and young adulthood, with up to five percent of young adults experiencing them. They peak between age 10 and 13 years, and thereafter become more likely in girls, but less likely in boys. Adult women experience more of them than adult men. There are no statistics on lifetime prevalence, but it's likely that all of us experience nightmares at some time or another.

Nightmares are a problem when they're so frequent that they disturb your sleep to the point of causing daytime sleepiness, or if you dwell on them during the day so that you become anxious or depressed.

Causes

Whether or not you experience nightmares is in part down to whether or not you have a genetic predisposition to them. If your parents or grandparents suffered from them, you're also more likely to. Some scientists have wondered if your waking personality makes you more susceptible – if you're more neurotic or thin-skinned during the day, are you more likely to have frightening, anxiety-fuelled dreams? As yet, we can't prove any direct association, but we do know that people who are more suggestible during the day (who have something that has been termed "boundary permeability"), and are more open and sensitive, do experience more nightmares than those who are, metaphorically speaking, thicker-skinned. Similarly, if you're a "coper" in wakefulness, you're more likely to be a coper in your dreams, too.

If genetics and personality don't provide all the answers, then what else triggers nightmares? Post Traumatic Stress Disorder (PTSD) provides us with further points of debate. Are the recurrent themes that appear in the nightmares of PTSD sufferers merely replays of a situation that occurred, or are they *actually* nightmares – frightening creations of the dream world? Are the two truly inseparable? As with so many things to do with sleep, we're still searching for the answers. Anecdotally, though, we know that children who've had a stressful or highly emotive experience – such as starting a new school, moving home or bullying – are more likely to also have nightmares; as are adults who have gone through bereavement, divorce or any other highly stressful life experience.

Finally, alcohol, drugs (both legal and illegal), a fever, and several other sleep disorders (including narcolepsy and night terrors) make us more prone to nightmares. Withdrawal from alcohol, caffeine or drugs are also risk factors for the disorder.

Treatments

The most supported treatment for nightmares is a process called "Image Rehearsal Therapy" (IRT). This treatment involves active engagement with the nightmare during the day. We do this by asking the patient to write a script of the nightmare, focusing on as much detail as possible, and then reading it back to minimize the emotions he or she associates with it, and also to see it through to a conclusion – for example, a victory, or an escape to safety and security. There's no set formula: it's up to you to work out how best to resolve your nightmare, and to rehearse that resolution so that if the nightmare, or one like it, recurs, you have the happy ending already planned out.

Recent studies reveal that lucid dreaming (see box, p.23) might offer successful treatment for nightmares. If you're able to lucid dream,

SLEEP SCIENCE

IS MODERN LIFE STEALING YOUR SLEEP?

It's popular these days to claim that our 24/7 lifestyle –
with practically unlimited access to information, shopping,
communication and so on – has brought about a level of constant
activity and, as a consequence, the worst levels of anxiety-related
sleep disorder of all time. I'm not sure that this is necessarily true.
In 1894, an article in the British Medical Journal claimed that
the increased pace of modern life at that time was the cause of
increased numbers of insomniacs. However, it went on to say that
with proper attention to dealing with stress, anxiety and workload
many people could in fact overcome their problems with sleep. The
same is as true now as it was then – perhaps the sources of stress
have changed, but we are just as capable as ever of changing our
responses to it, and in doing so of improving our sleep.

replay the nightmare during the daytime and work out a positive resolution. Repeat your scenario to yourself to embed it in your mind. Go
to bed as normal. If the nightmare or one like it recurs, while you're in
the dream you can become aware that you're dreaming, take control of
the action, and guide it to play out to its far less terrifying conclusion.

Lack of sleep can increase the likelihood and frequency of nightmares, so good sleep hygiene (see Chapter 3) is an essential form of
treatment. Practise the progressive muscle relaxation exercise in the
box on page 63, too – this exercise has been shown to reduce incidence
of nightmares in some people.

MENTAL DISORDER INSOMNIA

My first book examined the links between serotonin, sleep and mental
disorders. I found that there were links, but it wasn't clear how they
operated – and it's still not clear. I do now know, though, that there are

strong links between R sleep and depression. Periods of dreaming sleep come much earlier in the night for people who are depressed and are more evenly distributed throughout the night. Depressives also spend much less time in deep sleep. These anomalies normalize with the use of antidepressants, confirming that depression and sleep are linked. By 2020 we think that depression will be the second most disabling disorder among men and women. Any work we can do to unravel the links between sleep and depression is essential for our understanding not only of sleep but also of mental disorder in general.

Three main types of mental disorder are associated with insomnia (and other sleep disorders), of which depression is one; anxiety disorders and schizophrenia are the other two. In general, doctors believe that insomnia is a symptom of mental disorder, and that treating the disorder will give automatic relief from the insomnia. However, in order for doctors to recognize this kind of insomnia, a patient has to have found that the lack of sleep is affecting his or her life – in which case, it's important to tackle the insomnia as a separate entity, too.

I don't think it's as straightforward as simply that one causes the other. For example, sleep disturbance as a result of obstructive sleep apnoea (OSA; see pp.171–2) makes the sufferer almost twice as likely to suffer from depression but then those with depression are also more than one and a half times more likely to develop OSA. It's rather like the age-old question of which came first – the chicken or the egg?

Depression-related insomnia

Depression is subcategorized many times over, but in the first instance it's subdivided into "pure" depression (a permanent low mood) and bipolar depression (once called manic depression) – alternating periods of mania and low mood. Someone suffering from depression is likely to wake in the night and be unable to get back to sleep.

Interestingly, mania is characterized by very little sleep, and sleep deprivation or restriction may even trigger it. In a bizarre twist, sleep deprivation is used as an effective (albeit temporary) solution for pure depression, helping briefly to lift patients out of their depressed state.

Anxiety-related insomnia

Anxiety disorders (including post-traumatic stress disorder and general anxiety disorder) may make it hard for you to fall asleep. You may lie awake for many hours into the night waiting for sleep to come, but unable to quieten the stressed state of hyperarousal that characterizes your anxiety disorder. While it's important to adopt a rigorous approach to sleep hygiene to improve your sleep in these situations, it's also essential to deal with the source of the anxiety itself.

Schizophrenia-related insomnia

The relationship between schizophrenia and insomnia is complex and we're a long way off understanding how the two work together, partly because it's very hard to find schizophrenics who are unmedicated. Nonetheless, we do know that a period of insomnia can herald a schizophrenic episode – acting as a warning sign that the mind is out of kilter.

Treatments for mental disorder insomnia

If you've had insomnia for more than a month and, if relevant, it comes and goes with the ups and downs of your mental disorder, you should talk to your health practitioner about receiving treatment for the insomnia specifically. Although the insomnia and your mental disorder may be linked in some way, improving your sleep puts you in the strongest position for managing your other symptoms.

At home, optimize your sleep hygiene and then consider types of therapy – such as Cognitive Behavioural Therapy for Insomnia (see box, p.197), relaxation breathing exercises (box, p.71), and progressive muscle relaxation (see box, p.63) – that may help to improve your ability to sleep. However, owing to the delicate nature of mental disorder, I believe that it's inappropriate to offer generalized advice. I urge you to see your medical practitioner to receive individualized treatment – including guidance on self-help techniques – tailored to your own situation.

If self-help or a visit to a behavioural or cognitive psychologist can't improve your sleep, you may be prescribed medication to take only during the worst times of your sleep disorder.

CHAPTER 7

PILLS, POTIONS AND THERAPIES

By this point in the book, you know quite a lot about how sleep works, and how to improve your sleep hygiene to give you the best possible chance of having a good night's sleep. You also know about all the major insomnias and other sleep disorders. The final step is to bring together some of the therapies and medications available to you to support your efforts to take control of your sleep.

In this chapter I begin with some information about conventional medicines, including a table to introduce you to medications that you can buy over the counter and those your doctor may prescribe. Then you'll find advice on alternative therapies and natural medicines that have been shown to be beneficial to sleep. I'll explain what a sleep centre is and what happens if you visit one, and conclude with a whistlestop tour of some of the gadgets and gizmos that you can use at home to find out more about your sleep and how to improve it.

CONVENTIONAL MEDICINE

Conventional medicines are pharmaceutical drugs both prescribed by a medical doctor, appropriately qualified nurse or (in some countries) a pharmacist and "over-the-counter" (OTC) drugs. The latter are usually sold following a consultation with a pharmacist and bought directly off the shelf in a store. The laws covering the supply of medicines vary from country to country. Some of these differences may arise from cultural attitudes to taking medications to aid sleep.

A short history of sleeping pills

The proper term for sleeping pills is "hypnotics", derived from Hypnos, the Greek god of sleep, who is often depicted holding a poppy (the seeds of which give us opium, which in turn gives us morphine, a sedative). Since ancient times the search for natural or chemical sleep aids has, as you would expect, come a long way. In 1832, the German chemist Justus von Liebig synthesized the sedative chloral hydrate. Still in use today, chloral hyrdrate gained notoriety as a component of "Mickey Finn" – a dangerous combination of this sedative and alcohol.

In the mid-1800s the Prussian chemist Adolf von Baeyer synthesized compounds called barbiturates. These weren't used as hypnotics until the early 1900s, but then became the most common sleep aids right up until the 1970s. Barbiturates work, but they're extremely dangerous – overdoses can be (and have frequently been) fatal.

With this danger in mind, in the 1970s attention instead turned to benzodiazepines. Initially discovered in the 1950s, benzodiazepines came to the fore when it became clear that it was almost impossible to take a fatal overdose of them. However, the human body can develop a tolerance to these medications, meaning that their efficacy reduces the longer we take them. As we then need to take a higher dosage to achieve the same effects, addiction becomes a very real danger, followed by withdrawal symptoms when the hypnotics are stopped. In the 1990s, chemists synthesized the non-benzodiazepine "Z" drugs: zolpidem, zopiclone and zaleplon. Although these do have some risk of dependency, it is much lower than it is with benzodiazepines. Today, benzodiazepines and Z drugs remain the most widely prescribed drugs for insomnia.

Importantly, though, any drug taken to tackle a sleep disorder relieves the symptoms, but not the cause. While you may not know why you're suffering from insomnia, in order to find a long-term solution it's essential to live a lifestyle conducive to good sleep. Conventional medicine may help in the short term, as a coping strategy that enables you to put other things right, but it doesn't provide a safe, long-term solution. And, there's no "one size fits all" option – understanding the nature of your insomnia is important for getting your medication right, as well as for resolving your sleep problems altogether.

How do these drugs work?

In the body, GABA, a major neurochemical, attaches itself to certain nerve-cell receptors and affects how messages flow within those cells, inhibiting cell activity. Benzodiazepines and Z drugs – as well as barbiturates, chloral hydrate, and perhaps certain herbs (see p.200) – mimic GABA to have relaxing, anti-anxiety, anti-convulsive and amnesic effects. They also promote sleep. Older benzodiazepines that attach to the GABA receptors are described as "non-specific": they not only induce sleep, but also have, to some extent, all those other properties. Compounds that promote only sleep are "specific". Z drugs have similar effects to specific benzodiazepines, but are a separate class of drug.

What are the effects, side-effects and dangers?

All benzodiazepines and Z drugs can promote sleep. Some Z drugs increase deep sleep (see pp.19–22) and like the benzodiazepines improve the time it takes to fall asleep and the ability to fall back to sleep quickly if you wake in the night. Recent trials in the USA show that zolpidem, zaleplon and eszopiclone maintain their efficacy in the long term, making them less addictive.

When you stop taking any hypnotic, even after only a short time, you'll suffer a return to wakefulness, known as "rebound wakefulness" – your insomnia may appear worse, albeit only temporarily. Things are worse for long-term (chronic) users. Between 10 and 30 percent of long-term benzodiazepine users are physically dependent on the drug, and at least 50 percent will suffer from withdrawal *syndrome* when they cease medicating. The syndrome consists of anxiety, depression, nausea and perceptual changes, as well as rebound wakefulness. As a result, clinicians can prescribe these drugs only for severe insomnia and at the lowest dose possible for not more than four weeks.

Table 1 on the previous page lists the most commonly prescribed

TABLE 1: Common sleeping pills (generic not trade names). An asterisk (*) indicates that the breakdown products of the sleeping pills are also active (and extend the apparent half-life of the medication).

MEDICATION

Non-specific benzodiazepine	Usually prescribed for	Speed of action	Half-life (hours)	Common side-effects
Flurazepam	Insomnia	fast	48–120*	Risk of dependence; drowsiness or sedation; loss of muscle coordination; falling; behavioural changes (nervousness, confusion, aggression); loss of appetite
Temazepam	Insomnia	fast	8–20	
Nitrazepam	Insomnia	fast	15–40	
Loprazolam	Insomnia	slow	6–12	
Lormetazepam	Insomnia	slow	8–12	
Triazolam	Insomnia	very fast	2–6	
Quazepam	Insomnia	slow	39–73*	
Estazolam	Insomnia	fast	10–24	
Specific non-benzodiazepine				
Eszopiclone	Insomnia	fast	6	
Zaleplon	Insomnia	very fast	1	
Zolpidem	Insomnia	fast	1.5–2.4	
Zolpidem extended-release	Insomnia	fast	1.6–4.5	
Zopiclone	Insomnia	fast	3.5–6.5	
Non-specific non-benzodiazepine				
Chloral hydrate	Insomnia, alcohol withdrawal, anxiety	fast	7–10	
Clomethiazole	Severe insomnia in the elderly	fast	3.6–5	

hypnotics available in the UK or USA (some are available in only one country). Generally, sleeping pills are distinguished mainly by how quickly they can act and how long they stay in the brain and body. The time to reach maximum concentration in the blood is a good guide as to how quickly they act. The "half-life" is a measure of how long it takes the body to break down the drug – the shorter the time, the faster it's removed; the longer the half-life, the longer-lasting the effects.

If you have problems falling asleep, your doctor is likely to prescribe you a drug with a shorter half-life. If your issue is waking up in the night, your doctor may prescribe you a drug with a longer half-life. In the table "fast" means that the hypnotic is active within an hour.

Over-the-counter sleep medications and more

We think that up to 40 percent of people with insomnia self-medi-cate with non-prescription hypnotics bought in pharmacies. Although many of these medications contain compounds known to improve sleep, the fact that they're available without prescription tells you all you need to know about actually how effective they are for inducing sleep. Clinical trials for them usually involve small numbers of partici-pants, which means that results aren't as robust as they could be.

Table 2 on pages 194–5 lists many of the over-the-counter medica-tions that may aid sleep but that are not intended as hypnotics: most of them are to treat other medical disorders, but have soporific effects. Antihistamines, developed to treat allergies such as hay fever, have sedating effects that has added to their usage. Melatonin is a special case: I've given specific information about it on page 116. However, it's included in the table as it's now used in a formulation with the UK trademark "Circadin" for those over 55 and suffering from insomnia.

SLEEP CENTRES

Sleep centres are special clinics where experts can diagnose and treat sleep disorders. They are, in many countries, connected to hospital res-piratory departments. This is because sleep apnoea (see pp.171–4) has such strong links with other medical conditions. These centres concentrate on measuring the airflow through your nose, breathing effort and blood-oxygen levels. However, throughout the world, there are also now clinics specifically intended for dealing with the full spectrum of sleep disorders. A sleep centre might be suitable for you if:

- You have a persistent and ongoing problem with your sleep (such as an inability to sleep, broken sleep, snoring or other breathing-related disorders, or excessive daytime sleepiness).
- You've followed my methods for optimizing your sleep hygiene and yet see little improvement in your sleep quality.
- You don't want to begin relying on sleeping pills without first getting expert advice on the nature of your sleep problems.

What happens at a sleep centre?

A sleep centre will almost certainly send you a sleep diary (see pp.132–3) to fill in every night for (usually) two weeks before your appointment, as well as a questionnaire. What happens next depends on specialist analysis of your diary and your questionnaire answers.

- If your issues might be to do with your biological clock, you may be given an actigraph to wear. This monitors your levels of activity and rest over the course of 24 hours.
- If you have suspected sleep apnoea or other physiological causes for your sleep issues, you may be given an oximeter (a clip that attaches usually to your finger) to measure oxygen and haemoglobin levels in your blood, a nose clip to chart your air-flow and a chest band to assess your breathing.
- If your sleep disorder needs further investigation, you may be given a full polysomnography examination. This is the main diagnostic tool at all sleep centres and will require you to stay overnight at the centre (see below).

Monitoring your sleep at a sleep centre

At a sleep centre you'll be given a room and connected up to wiring that will measure your sleep. Many people worry that they won't actually be able to sleep in these clinical conditions. However, with so much excessive sleepiness already clocked up, and the security of

TABLE 2: Non-hypnotic sleep aids (over-the-counter medications)

Sedating antidepressants		Speed of action	Half-life (hours)	Insomnia dosage (mg)	Common side-effects
Amitriptyline	Depression	medium	10–100	10–100	Drowsiness; dry mouth; blurred vision; constipation
Doxepin	Depression, anxiety	fast	10–50	1–25	
Mirtazapine	Depression	fast	20–40	7.5–30	
Trimipramine	Depression	medium	15–40	25–100	
Trazodone	Depression	fast	7–15	25–150	
Antipsychotics					
Olanzapine	Schizophrenia, mania	slow	20–54	2.5–20	Feeling sleepy or tired; gaining weight; high cholesterol; high blood sugar
Quetiapine	Schizophrenia, depression, mania	fast	7	25–200	
Anticonvulsants					
Gabapentin	Epilepsy, pain	slow	5–9	100–900	Drowsiness; restlessness and irritability; confusion and dizziness; nausea, vomiting, loss of appetite, and stomach pain; uncontrollable eye movements (nystagmus); gum disease (gingivitis); itching, fever, and a rash that looks like measles (sensitivity reaction); weight gain
Pregabalin	Fibromyalagia, epilepsy, pain	fast	4.5–7	50–300	
Tiagabine	Epilepsy	fast	8	2–16	

Melatonin and melatonin receptor agonists					
Melatonin	Hormone supplement (prescribed in the UK; OTC in the USA)	fast	0.6–1	0.3.–1	May interact with blood pressure medications and increase symptoms in diabetes, depression and seizure disorders
Melatonin SR (*Circadin*)	Depression	fast			
Ramelteon	Insomnia (US)	fast	0.8–2	0.7–0.95	Drowsiness; dizziness; headache; low energy
Antihistamines					
Diphenhydramine	Allergy, insomnia (OTC)	slow	5–11	2–2.5	Dry mouth; drowsiness; dizziness; nausea and vomiting; restlessness or moodiness (in some children); difficulty urinating or inability to urinate; blurred vision; confusion
Doxylamine	Insomnia (OTC)	fast	10–12	1.5–2.5	
Promethazine	Insomnia	slow			
Other Drugs					
Sodium oxybate	Narcolepsy	very fast	0.3–1.2	0.5–0.8	Depression, throat Irritation; sinus irritation and congestion; infection; problems with bladder control; confusion

knowing that you're in the process of finding out what's going on so that you can finally take control of your sleep, you'll probably have one of the best nights you've had in a long time. Certainly, in most cases, sleep at a sleep centre is no worse than it is at home.

Overnight monitoring involves three sets of basic wiring. First, you'll need to have multiple electrodes (each smaller than a penny) glued to your face and scalp. These measure your brainwaves, eye movements and chin-muscle tone (during dreaming sleep the chin muscles become active). They provide all the information a sleep expert needs to map your journey through sleep's main stages.

Technicians attach the electrodes to your scalp using a special glue. You won't need to have any hair shaved and in my experience you'll be combing glue out of your hair for a while after the sleep study!

Second, the centre needs to measure your breathing and oxygen levels. This may involve sensors on your nose (airflow) and fingers (blood-oxygen levels), and in chest straps (to record your breathing movements, including how deeply you breathe and how often).

Finally, as limb movements can disturb your sleep, further electrodes will be attached to your legs. You may have electrodes placed on any other part of your body that might be causing a problem, too.

All the wires connect up to a junction box somewhere near the head of your bed, in such a way that you're able to turn over during the night. There may also be some camera equipment set up in the room, which will take video recordings of you as you sleep.

Diagnosis and treatment

Armed with such specific information about how you sleep, experts can usually work out fairly quickly why your sleep is not restful. They can then recommend an individualized treatment, using techniques best suited to your situation. These might include medical treatments, such as an operation to remove your adenoids or tonsils or excess tissue in your throat if you're suffering from a breathing disorder, as well as treatments such as clinical hypnotherapy, which can help with overcoming certain insomnias and parasomnias; or Cognitive Behavioural Therapy for Insomnia (see box, p.197), which can help to

SLEEP SCIENCE

COGNITIVE BEHAVIOURAL THERAPY FOR INSOMNIA (CBT-I)

Throughout the world sleep experts use CBT-I as a main treatment for insomnia. The objective is to modify the negative behaviours that lead to insomnia and to learn how to reduce the number of intrusive thoughts you have that inhibit your ability to sleep, as well as the anxiety you associate with sleeping.

As a first step, a therapist will ask you to keep a diary of your thoughts – whether they're related to sleep, or any of the other things going on in your life – and your sleep. Once you've identified problematic thought patterns that might be interfering with your sleep, you can challenge them by replacing them with accurate beliefs (for example, changing a thought such as "I can't cope if I don't get a good night's sleep" to "I'll have a tired day if I don't get a good night's sleep, but I'll sleep better the following night to make up for it.") and more realistic attitudes. Your statements may need to be related to a specific aspect of your sleep hygiene. For example, if you're making negative associations with your bed, you'll need to change your attitude so that you positively associate the bed with sleep. A therapist will help to show you how.

In general, positive statements about sleep help to give you reasons to start believing again in your ability to sleep. Simple statements such as "sleep is easy" or "I can sleep" can have a powerful effect when repeated over and over, every day, rewiring your brain to believe in sleep as something that comes naturally.

Some therapists use other psychotherapy techniques, such as distraction training and dedicated "worry time", but whatever the methodology, the basic principle is the same – to turn all negative associations with sleep into sleep-inducing positive ones.

change the way you think about your sleep.

COMPLEMENTARY MEDICINE

Covering all non-conventional medicine, complementary medicine includes natural treatments such as herbalism or natural supplements, non-Western medical systems such as Traditional Chinese Medicine and Ayurvedic medicine, as well as those that have been more recently developed, such as modern-day energy treatments.

Even as a scientist, I do not discount the power of the mind and of nature. However, in many cases there's been little scientific rigour in the testing of whether or not complementary therapies have any worth in the sphere of sleep medicine. In order to recommend a treatment, I do need to know that it's been scrutinized in a scientific way.

Amazingly, rigorous testing hasn't extended to the scientific assessment of massage, osteopathy, homeopathy and aromatherapy. This doesn't mean that these therapies don't work to promote sleep, just that there's no available evidence that they do. There have been, though, sufficient studies to evaluate acupuncture and acupressure; the herbs kava (*Piper methysticum*) and valerian root (*Valeriana officinalis*) individually and in combination and a combination of valerian root and hops (*Humulus lupulus*); supplementation of tryptophan (an amino acid); and the mind–body practices of tai chi and yoga.

What were the outcomes?

The practices of acupressure, yoga and tai chi have shown positive support for dealing with insomnia, with acupressure coming out best. This involves a practitioner applying finger pressure to classic acupuncture points related to sleep (see box, opposite). Treatments generally last between six and eight weeks.

The mind–body therapies of yoga and tai chi had beneficial effects over a period of weeks. My favourite is yoga, as the discipline has three components that I think are fundamental to improving the quality of sleep. First, yoga involves various breathing techniques (see box, p.71 for one of them), which help to reduce heart rate and lower anxiety.

ACUPRESSURE FOR SLEEP

As part of your wind-down routine, try the following acupressure exercise to stimulate the sleep-sensitive acupressure points.

1. Use your thumb to press gently but firmly on the point between your eyebrows at the top of your nose, where there's a slight indentation. Hold for 20 seconds, then release briefly, and repeat the pressure twice more.

2. Sit upright on the end of your bed and put your right foot across your left knee, supporting it underneath with your left hand. Keep your left foot flat on the floor. Find the slight indent on the top of your right foot between your big toe and your second toe. Use your right thumb to press firmly down on this point, until you feel a slight discomfort. Hold for 20 seconds, then release briefly, and repeat the pressure twice more.

3. Still supporting your right foot, find the point just below the nail on the upper side of your second toe. Using the thumb and forefinger of your right hand, gently squeeze the toe, applying pressure to this point. Hold for 20 seconds, release briefly, and repeat the pressure twice more.

Second, it encourages strength and flexibility, which are essential for releasing tension in the muscles and in this way helping to prevent aches and pains that might disturb sleep. And third, yoga encourages mindfulness – being fully present in the moment and so distracting the mind from any thoughts about not being able to sleep.

Finally, the results with tryptophan were inconclusive, although anecdotal evidence suggests that taking supplements of this amino acid may be of help. Herbal remedies need a little more explanation.

Herbal remedies

Of the herbs that have been rigorously tested, only valerian root has come close to standing up to scrutiny as a sleep treatment (see box, opposite for a valerian bedtime drink). Historically, though, many herbs have been put forward as treatments to help combat sleeplessness. I've listed these below, but note that these haven't been rigorously tested for their sleep-promoting qualities.

- Garden camomile (*Anthemus nobile*) and German camomile (*Matricaria chamomilla*) for anxiety and insomnia.
- Jamaican dogwood (*Piscidia erythrina*) for pain-related sleeplessness.
- Lady's slipper (*Cypripedium pubescens*) for sleeplessness associated with anxiety.
- Lavender (*Lavendula officinalis*) possibly for sleeplessness in the elderly and for its potential antidepressant effects.
- Passion flower (*Passiflora incarnata*) for anxiety and insomnia.
- Peppermint (*Mentha* x *piperita*) for sleeplessness when you have a cold.
- Wild lettuce (*Lactuca virosa*) for insomnia (and reputedly used for this since ancient times).
- St John's wort (*Hypericum perforatum*) for its potential to improve depression-related insomnia.

GADGETS, GIZMOS AND THE WORLD WIDE WEB

For most of the life of sleep medicine, gadgets and gizmos have been the province of research laboratories and sleep centres (see pp.192–8). Now, versions of these technologies are available for us to download or to buy and use in the home.

Devices are broadly those that track your sleep (trackers), help you get to sleep (mollifiers) and wake you up (grizzlies). Internet websites can provide a personalized sleep service to help you to monitor your sleep and find advice that's unique to your own sleep situation.

SLEEP THERAPY

COOL VALERIAN ROOT INFUSION

Use the following "recipe" to make a valerian root infusion. However, please check with a qualified herbalist that the herb is not contraindicated for you first. Have one cup of the infusion as part of your pre-sleep routine every night for up to six weeks. Break for two weeks, then resume for up to another six weeks if necessary.

Crush 1 tsp of valerian root in a pestle and mortar and soak it in one cup of cool, filtered water for up to 24 hours. Strain the infusion and drink cold.

Trackers

These range from those that are essentially simple diaries, recording the time you go to sleep and wake up, and asking for information about the quality of your sleep; to highly sophisticated devices such as the Zeo (see box, p.202). Many trackers are available as straight-forward smartphone apps, and many are free to download. Inevitably, some are more useful than others, but generally I recommend those that disconnect your phone from the network and shut down your connection to your Wi-Fi during the night. In this way you can make sure that you won't be disturbed by late-night communications, but you can still use all the features of the app.

Somewhere between these simple apps and the Zeo lie trackers that measure your movement during sleep and match that to the phases of sleep. An accelerometer built into the app means that, once down-loaded, the app allows your smartphone to monitor how much you're moving about during the night and also works out when, once you've had your sleep quota, you're in the lightest phase of sleep so that you can wake feeling most refreshed. If you don't have a smartphone, you can find similar devices that you wear on your wrist.

All these devices have the advantage of allowing you to track your sleep more accurately than you could by simply relying upon your

SLEEP SCIENCE

THE ZEO

Of all the devices on the market, the Zeo™ is the most remarkable. It both records and analyzes sleep via two small units: a headband with three silverized pads and a clip-on sensor, and a bedside unit that tracks data via a Wi-Fi link from the headband.

To use the Zeo all you have to do is to put on the headband as you turn out the lights to sleep. The bedside unit displays whether or not the connection is OK. In the morning, you put the headband and sensor on your bedside unit, which automatically ends the recording and charges the sensor for the following night.

The Zeo uses a memory card to store the data about your sleep, and you can use the card to upload the information to *myzeo.com* (or *.co.uk*), which will decipher the amount of light, deep and dreaming sleep you get each night you wear the device. The sleep diary function enables you to input information about your caffeine, alcohol and exercise levels to provide the basis for a personalized coaching program accessed through the website.

The Zeo is not a medical device and it can't replace the level of insight you would receive at a sleep centre. However, it does have huge potential. Chronic insomnia probably arises from repeated acute insomnia. The Zeo is well placed to identify causes of poor sleep so that you can help prevent sleeplessness turning into insomnia. Its greatest potential, though, lies in the way in which it can identify how sleep affects your daytime performance. If you wake up in the morning, feel you've slept well and yet don't then function at your best, the Zeo can show you whether or not something went wrong with your deep or dreaming sleep. If it did, you know you need to take steps to improve your sleep in order that you can improve your daytime functioning.

memory of what happened overnight. In addition, as many of them link to websites that provide fully blown sleep diary functions, you can very quickly build up an accurate picture of your sleep quality and under what circumstances you sleep best.

Mollifiers

Your bedroom should be a place kept as technology-free as possible. However, mollifiers aim to improve your sleep hygiene, so they're an exception to the rule. For example, if noise is keeping you awake, you can buy devices that play white noise, or neutral or pleasant sounds. Some come with earphones that go inside your ears, but I think those with a headband are more comfortable. In addition, those that detect when you've fallen asleep and then turn off automatically help to prevent continuous sound from disturbing your slumber. See pp.50–54 for more information on noise-reducing gadgets.

Nightlights and dawnlights (that simulate dawn to wake you up naturally) also fall under the category of mollifiers (see p.50).

Grizzlies

If you don't wake up naturally – as you reach the end of a sleep cycle after a full, refreshing night – you're probably using an alarm (or have young children). Grizzlies are, essentially, alarm clocks. They vary in their gentleness and it's up to you to decide whether you prefer a gentle rousing into the day or to wake up with a great clang. Personally, I like the idea of the alarm mat. You place it at the head of your bed and have to get your feet out and stand on it to turn it off – this means there's no danger of simply ignoring the alarm or switching it to snooze without moving more than an arm.

If you and your partner need to wake up at different times, you could try a novel device that consists of two little rings – one for each of you – and a single dock through which you can programme each ring individually to vibrate at a certain time. When you go to bed, you each put your ring on the end of one of your forefingers. Your ring vibrates silently at the time you want to wake up, in theory waking you, but not your partner – or vice versa, depending upon who needs

SLEEP CLINIC

I often have to work late at my computer and I know this is affecting my sleep. Are there any gadgets that can help?

If working late at a screen is completely unavoidable, you could try downloading a program such as "Flux" that automatically adjusts the brightness of your screen to mimic the ambient light in your office or study. Computer screens are generally programmed to assume you're working in daylight. At night this can dazzle your eyes, making it hard to switch off when you go to bed. While dimming the screen using the brightness keys can help, online programs can adjust the screen so that it doesn't simply get greyed out (and in the process becomes actually quite hard to focus on), but instead mimics the light you have around you. So, if you tell the program you're working in an office with halogen light, it works out that it needs to adjust your screen from daylight to halogen light as darkness falls. The idea is that you aren't bombarded with lux from your screen late into the night, which means that your eyes feel less achey and dazzled when it's time to go to bed.

to get up first. The vibration stops when you put the ring back on the dock. Of course, whoever gets up first is still going to need to creep out of bed and get ready very quietly!

Finally, for some fun and to get your morning exercise in, you could try the alarm clock that comes as part of a dumbbell. You have to do the "repetitions" to stop the alarm from ringing!

Links and references for all these gadgets are given on page 208.

The World Wide Web

Since the time I wrote my first sleep help website ten years ago, and since the Sleep Assessment and Advisory Service (of which I'm a director) began providing online as well as phone advice, there's been a huge expansion in the numbers of sites providing information on insomnia, its causes and its cures. A search I just recently made for "insomnia help" gave more than 78,100,000 websites to look at!

The growth of sleep medicine as a serious science in both the USA and Europe has led to lots of websites providing high-quality information, albeit all along the same lines. Now, simply through your computer, you can have a consultation or therapeutic session using video-communication software, such as Skype or Google Hangouts. Furthermore, there are lots of self-assessment programs and automated programs that deliver Cognitive Behavioural Therapy for Insomnia (see box, p.197). The Mood Gym is one of the earliest and best-established of these, but there's also now Living Life to the Full, devised by Dr Chris Williams of Glasgow University. You can find the links for both these in the Resources section of the book on page 208. In addition, there are plenty of websites that deliver advice on how to beat depression and overcome anxiety, and even one specifically intended to overcome insomnia (again, see p.208 for links).

You'll find overlap on most sites (depression and mood sites cover insomnia, too). Most cover topics such as emotional intelligence, managing stress, relaxation techniques, coping with difficult events, improving self-esteem and relationships, problem solving, time management, positive thinking and, of course, sleep management.

The opportunity for taking control of your life – and your sleep – has never been greater or more accessible. All the websites listed on my resources page, and a wealth of others, can help you learn about what in your life could be affecting your sleep, and many offer sound advice on how to make effective changes that could change your sleep – and your wakefulness – for good.

CONCLUSION

Over the pages of this book, you'll have gleaned that sleep medicine, still in its relative infancy, has a long way to go before we fully understand what happens to our bodies and brains during the hours of the night. Nonetheless, I hope I've been able to unravel some of the secrets of your sleeping life so that you can make changes that enable you to fall asleep easily, sleep soundly, and wake up refreshed. In summary, here are my top five pointers for getting the best out of your sleep:

- First and foremost, optimize your sleep hygiene. I've said it often, but good sleep hygiene really is the key to healthy sleep.
- Make sure that you take steps to reduce anxiety and increase relaxation in your life. Stressed people don't sleep well.
- If you think you might have a sleep disorder, investigate it as soon as possible – don't wait, hoping it will pass: that's how minor disorders become insomnias.
- If your first go at self-help doesn't work, think about visiting your medical practitioner or other healthcare professional to check that a sinister disorder isn't causing the problem. Prescription medications are available only through a medical practitioner, some others through a pharmacist, others off the shelf in a pharmacy, and others still at the supermarket. However, remember that any medication is only ever masking the underlying problem.
- Finally, believe in your ability to sleep. What we still have to learn about sleep does not change the fact that sleep is a natural, necessary state for well-being.

RESOURCES

If you'd like to get in touch to ask me about your own sleep experiences, or if you'd like to read about the latest news and research I've been involved in, please visit my websites: **www.sleepspecialist.co.uk** and **www.neuronic.com**

For specific information or products, you might like to try:

Sleep, behavioural and relaxation therapies

Beating the blues:
www.beatingthe blues.co.uk

Fear Fighter: www.fearfighter.com

Sleepio: www.sleepio.com

The Mood Gym:
moodgym.anu.edu.au/welcom

Living Live to the Full:
www.llttf.com

Dream On: www.dreamonapp.com

Jet lag calculator

www.britishairways.com/travel/
drsleep/public/en_gb?
cookiesAccepted=existpop

Gadgets and gizmos

Nighmo: www.nighmo.com

The Zeo: www.myzeo.co.uk or
www.myzeo.com

Alarm clock mat:
www.yankodesign.com/
2007/06/19/carpet-alarm-clock

Two-ring alarm clock:
www.yankodesign.com/
2007/07/10/alarming-ring/

The dumbbell alarm clock and dawn simulation alarm clock are available from online retailers such as Amazon.

Light box: http://www.sadbox.co.uk

Sleep disorder centres

UK: www.sleeping.org.uk

USA: www.sleepfoundation.org

INDEX